Paleo Desserts

FOR DUMMIES®

A Wiley Brand

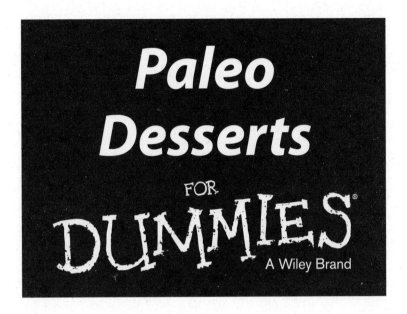

Paleo Desserts

FOR DUMMIES®
A Wiley Brand

by Adriana Harlan

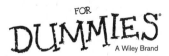

FOR DUMMIES®
A Wiley Brand

Paleo Desserts **For Dummies**®

Published by
John Wiley & Sons, Inc.,
111 River Street, Hoboken,
NJ 07030-5774
www.wiley.com

Copyright © 2015 by John Wiley & Sons, Inc., Hoboken, New Jersey

Published simultaneously in Canada

For general information on our other products and services, please contact our Customer Care Department within the U.S. at 877-762-2974, outside the U.S. at 317-572-3993, or fax 317-572-4002.

For technical support, please visit www.wiley.com/techsupport.

Wiley publishes in a variety of print and electronic formats and by print-on-demand. Some material included with standard print versions of this book may not be included in e-books or in print-on-demand. If this book refers to media such as a CD or DVD that is not included in the version you purchased, you may download this material at http://booksupport.wiley.com. For more information about Wiley products, visit www.wiley.com.

Library of Congress Control Number: 2014958562

ISBN: 97-811-1902280-0

ISBN 97-811-1902282-4 (ePub); ISBN 97-811-1902283-1 (PDF)

Manufactured in the United States of America

10 9 8 7 6 5 4 3 2 1

Contents at a Glance

Table of Contents

Introduction

Making changes to your diet and lifestyle is imperative for regaining a healthy body and the life you love. Living Paleo nourishes your mind, body, and soul, and it's much more than a diet. It's a template that guides you toward your healthiest and most-balanced self. When you go Paleo, you learn to eat whole foods designed for your own unique body. You also learn to manage stress and make time for sleep and exercise. These changes transform your body and life, giving you health, happiness, energy, and vitality.

What you don't do is give up on indulging your natural craving for treats. The genetic makeup of the human body has changed very little from our hunter-gatherer ancestors, and even they had a sweet tooth. Therefore, the only nutritional approach that helps you stay strong, lean, and healthy is to consume a diet rich in essential minerals and vitamins and free of processed modern foods. *Paleo Desserts For Dummies* helps you do just that without depriving yourself.

Whether your goal is to lose weight, look your best, improve your family's health, or simply discover the healthy alternatives to sugar- and chemical-laden junk foods, *Paleo Desserts For Dummies* is the resource you've been waiting for. In this book, I give you my best cooking tips and healthy Paleo dessert recipes so you can enjoy life more without having to deprive yourself of your favorite foods.

About This Book

Paleo Desserts For Dummies is a reference guide as well as a cookbook. Transitioning to the Paleo diet and lifestyle is simple; you may already be following many of its principles. Choosing unprocessed and nutritious ingredients to make savory desserts also help you stay focused and motivated.

This book introduces you to the basic principles of the Paleo diet and lifestyle. You discover how to stock your kitchen with real foods and natural ingredients to make sweets and treats. I explain the basics of Paleo baking and list some essential kitchen tools to make cooking easy and enjoyable. Oh, and you get 11 yummy chapters with more than 100 Paleo dessert recipes, including cakes, pies, cookies, brownies, ice creams, breads, muffins, candies, jams, nut butters, and other delectable sweet sauces. Some chapters even focus on special holiday celebrations such as Thanksgiving, Halloween, Christmas, and Hanukkah.

I've also included some information in shaded sidebars; these bits are interesting but not essential to your success as a Paleo baker/chocolatier. If you just want the down-and-dirty essentials, you can skip the sidebars, as well as anything marked with a Technical Stuff icon.

Finally, I've used a few conventions in the recipes:

- ✔ All temperatures are in degrees Fahrenheit. You can find Fahrenheit to Celsius converters online.

- ✔ All coconut oil is unrefined. Goods made with unrefined coconut oil may have a slight coconut taste; if the flavor bothers you, you can use refined coconut oil.

- ✔ When I refer to "Paleo-friendly chocolate," I mean chocolate that's at least 70 percent cacao and is soy-free.

- ✔ I use the scoop-and-level approach for measuring dry ingredients and measure liquid ingredients in dry measuring utensils, which may different from techniques you've used previously. Chapter 3 has details on using these methods.

A final note: You may find the recipes in this cookbook extremely delicious, but they're still treats, so don't overindulge.

Icons Used in This Book

Throughout this book, I have included helpful icons that highlight key concepts and information about the Paleo lifestyle and Paleo dessert-making:

This icon points you to helpful cooking suggestions and information that — when applied — creates changes that result in a healthier, happier you!

The Warning icon is a signal for potential pitfalls that may trip you up, either in Paleo baking or in your overall Paleo lifestyle.

Whenever you see this icon, keep an eye out for important information you should always keep stashed in your memory.

The Technical Stuff icon flags text that's interesting but nonessential. You don't have to read it to benefit from this book, but I recommend you do anyway!

Foolish Assumptions

As I wrote this book, I made a few assumptions about you, dear reader; if any of the following applies to you, this book is for you:

- ✔ You want to be healthy and feel your best without having to give up sweets and treats.
- ✔ You want to discover a world of delicious, healthy desserts that are easy to make.
- ✔ You want to get off the sugar-rush roller coaster.
- ✔ You love baking but want to discover how to bake with healthy, unprocessed ingredients.
- ✔ You're new to the Paleo approach to health and want to know more.

Beyond the Book

Beyond all the recipes and information in this book, I have reserved some special goodies that you can access anytime for free on the web. Check out the eCheat Sheet at www.dummies.com/cheatsheet/paleodesserts and the bonus content at www.dummies/extras/paleodesserts I created just for you to help you get started living a healthy lifestyle and creating delicious Paleo desserts.

While you're online, come say hi to me on my blog, ask me questions, and check out all the new dessert recipes I create at www.livinghealthywith chocolate.com.

Where to Go from Here

This book is organized in such a way that you can read the chapters in any order that you prefer. Feel free to look over the table of contents to find specific subjects of interest or use the index to look up specific keywords and information.

Consider starting with Chapter 3 if you want to get a handle on the nuts and bolts of Paleo dessert-making, the different natural ingredients available, and the importance of measuring those ingredients. Then move over to Chapter 2 for info on stocking your Paleo baking pantry. You also may want to just skip straight to Parts II and III and check out all the dessert recipes available, which start with Chapter 4 and go through Chapter 14.

And don't skip Chapters 15 and 16. You get all kinds of tips and tricks for making Paleo desserts, which make your life easier and your sweet treats more yummy.

If you're not sure where to start and you're new to Paleo, my advice is to read the chapters in order. This approach gives you the knowledge you need to get started living a healthy Paleo lifestyle while also adopting its nutritional principles. Reading through the beginning chapters helps you understand why this lifestyle is so effective in improving your health and quality of life.

Part I

Reaping the Benefits of Paleo Desserts

getting started with

Benefits of Paleo Desserts

Visit www.dummies.com for great Dummies content online.

In This Part . . .

- ✔ Learn the fundamental principles of the Paleo diet and find out why this is a lifestyle, not just a diet.

- ✔ Get an insight into which essential macronutrients humans depend on to sustain a healthy body, and which toxic foods to avoid.

- ✔ Discover why food quality plays an important role in further creating health and wellness.

- ✔ Find out why the Paleo diet goes way beyond eating healthy foods and how the lifestyle choices you make help you achieve positive results.

- ✔ Get advice on how to clear your kitchen of toxic foods and restock your shelves with wholefoods as well as Paleo-approved baking ingredients.

- ✔ Discover how sweets can be part of a healthy diet, and get my best tips and tricks for making Paleo desserts.

Chapter 1

What is Paleo?

. . . .

In This Chapter

▶ Understanding the foundations and history of the Paleo lifestyle

▶ Identifying the stars of a Paleo diet

▶ Recognizing the benefits of feeding the body with proper nutrition

▶ Enjoying sweets with a Paleo approach

. . . .

*T*he Paleo diet has become very popular worldwide because it's less of a diet and more of a lifestyle that you can follow without calorie restrictions. This lifestyle emphasizes eating natural, wholesome foods that feed the body with proper nutrition. Living Paleo helps you get to know your own body better and achieve optimal health, preventing diseases, healing inflammation, and boosting youthful energy.

Avoiding harmful ingredients and choosing high-quality foods (from organic produce to pasture-raised animal proteins) transforms lives, and thousands of people are reaping the benefits of eating this way. Unlike fad diets, the Paleo diet is quite simple; it gives you a template to choose nutritious foods while making you aware of the foods that your body can't efficiently digest and absorb. Because Paleo isn't a restrictive diet, you don't have to give up eating your favorite foods — including sweets and treats! You may just have to approach making them a little differently. The dessert recipes in this book follow the primal nutritional blueprint and are made with truly natural ingredients. This chapter introduces some fundamental Paleo principles.

Picking Up the Basics of Eating Paleo

The *Paleo diet,* also known as the *caveman* or *primal diet,* is based on the simple nutritional principle that you should consume only the foods your body was designed to eat. It attempts to emulate the whole, unprocessed nature of a hunter-gatherer diet by eating foods rich in nutrients.

The fundamental idea behind this concept is the fact that the human genome has changed very little in the last 40,000 years — only about 0.02 percent, according to studies. It has been 12,000 years since the onset of the agricultural era, which is a drop in the evolutionary bucket, but long enough for some people to develop at least a degree of tolerance to agricultural-based foods. The degree to which individuals can tolerate agricultural-based foods may depend on a variety of factors, including ancestral background, age, and health status. It's important to consider that the last few generations have grown up on heavily processed foods and with other circumstances that have not fostered good gut health (a lack of breastfeeding or exposure to antibiotics and other drugs, for example). The result is that many people today already have a compromised gut that reduces tolerance to agricultural-based foods. In addition, the characteristics of the food and proper preparation methods come into play, as modern grains have been bred to be much different from the grains consumed even 200 years ago and traditional preparation techniques that make grains safer to consume have been lost in our culture.

The foods you eat therefore manipulate how your genes function and perform. Your genes are a living being, always adapting and growing. Premature aging and other conditions most people chalk up to bad genes are often actually the result of genes that have changed because you didn't supply your cells with proper nutrients. The good news is that the nutrients an individual consumes can influence whether certain genes are turned on or off.

For thousands of years, our hunter-gatherer ancestors depended on essential *nutrients* to sustain life. Traditional cultures throughout history recognized the need to consume nutrient-dense foods in order to support health and encourage fertility The Okinawans and the Mediterraneans, for example, knew by careful observation that eating certain foods was necessary to ensure the community's long-term survival.

These essential nutrients are far different from what conventional wisdom considers optimal today. For decades, the party line in the Western world has been that health means exercising more and eating fewer calories, less fat, and more grain-based carbs. But a wealth of scientific research supports the strong correlation between the recommended consumption of industrialized foods and the epidemics of diabetes, cancer, and cardiovascular disease you see today. The following sections break down what should and shouldn't be on your Paleo menu to be fit, lean and strong like your hunter-gatherer ancestors.

Filling up on Paleo-friendly proteins, carbs, and fats

When you adopt a Paleo lifestyle, you no longer eat what's known as the Standard American Diet (which is full of processed junk). Instead, your focus turns to eating whole foods from high-quality proteins, carbohydrates, and fat, including meat, poultry, fish, eggs, non-starchy vegetables and fruits, nuts, and seeds. In the following sections, I take a closer look at each of these nutrients.

Protein

Protein is essential for every cell in the body. It fuels the body to support strong muscles and healthy bones and build and repair tissue. Animal proteins provide complete sources of amino acids that the body can't produce. The most suitable sources of protein are from healthy, pasture-raised animals that didn't receive antibiotics, hormones, or genetically modified feed. Beef, lamb, pork, seafood, and raw dairy are easy to absorb and supply the body with protein as well as healthy fats, vitamin D, and selenium. Game animals such as goats, rabbits, wild boar, and venison (deer) are also good options. Eggs supply the body with omega-3 fatty acids and key micronutrients such as vitamins A, D, and B. (Head to the later section "Fat" for more on omega-3s and other healthy fats.)

Purchase the highest-quality animal protein you can find. Meats should be labeled as *organic, grass-fed,* and *grass-finished.* Poultry and eggs should be *free-range* or *pastured.* Fish and other seafood should be *wild-caught.* Dairy should be *organic, grass-fed, unpasteurized* (raw), and *non-homogenized.*

Carbohydrates

Studies indicate that on average, traditional hunter-gatherer societies ate between 3 to 50 percent of their total calories from carbohydrates depending on the latitude at which these societies lived. But the types of carbohydrates they consumed were very different than what health authorities recommend today. For thousands of years — until the Industrial Revolution — humans ate whole-food sources of carbohydrates from fruits, starchy tubers and plants, seaweed, nuts, and honey. In contrast, the Standard American Diet today consists mostly of highly processed and refined carbohydrates, such as the grains and sugars found in breads, pasta, cereals, pastries, and more.

Assuming you have a healthy metabolism, the bulk of your daily intake of carbohydrates should between 15 to 30 percent. If you are trying to lose weight or have blood sugar problems, aim to get between 10 to 15 percent of total calories from carbohydrates daily. Non-starchy vegetables can be eaten freely throughout the day assuming you can digest them well. Two to five servings of fruits is recommended daily unless you have blood sugar issues or are trying to lose weight, which in case you should choose to eat low-sugar fruits like berries. Eating starchy plants is recommended in the range of two to four servings daily unless you are trying to lose weight or have blood sugar problems.

Tracing the history of the lowfat lie

Health authorities and the media have demonized eating fats for years, telling you it makes you fat and causes heart disease, all based on flawed research done by Ancel Keys and his *Seven* Countries study that started in 1947. Keys was a member of the nutrition committee at the American Heart Association, and he went on to the U.S. Senate to promote his hypothesis that saturated fat causes heart disease. That's when the low-fat craze started and people began consuming highly processed vegetable oils such as soybean and canola oil (margarine) and a diet high in refined carbohydrates. It was during this time that the occurrence of diabetes, obesity, cancer, and gallstones skyrocketed. Eating a lowfat diet high in refined carbohydrates changes the efficiency at which your cells transport blood sugar, proteins, hormones, bacteria, viruses, and tumor-causing agents through your body, thus leading to these modern-day diseases.

Here are some nutrient-dense, wholefood Paleo carbohydrates:

- ✓ **Non-starchy vegetables:** Asparagus, broccoli, Brussels sprouts, bok choy, cabbage, cauliflower, eggplant, mushrooms, onions, leeks, garlic, peppers, zucchini, carrots, tomatoes, and seaweed

- ✓ **Leafy greens:** Collard greens, kale, Swiss chard, mustard greens, lettuce, spinach, parsley, and arugula

- ✓ **Starchy tubers and root vegetables:** Sweet potatoes, plantains, yams, yucca, tapioca, arrowroot, squash, and pumpkin

- ✓ **Fruits:** Berries, cherries, apples, pears, grapefruit, apricots, peaches, and figs

Fat

Consuming fat is not only essential for your health but also critical for cell construction, nerve function, digestion, hormonal balance, and vitamin absorption. For example, the human brain is composed of 70 percent fat. Over the course of millions of years, humans depended on fat to survive and evolve.

Fats aren't all the same, and they aren't all bad for you; each type of fat affects the body in a different way. The following list details the healthy fats you can make part of your Paleo lifestyle:

- ✓ **Long-chain saturated fats**: *Long-chain saturated fats* make up 75 to 80 percent of fatty acids in most cells in the human body. When you eat foods containing this type of fat, your body stores the fat and converts it into energy efficiently and without toxic by-products. These healthy saturated fats can be found in fattier cuts of pastured-raised meats such as beef, lamb, and pork, as well as raw/pastured dairy. If you have a healthy metabolism, eating saturated fats with every meal will give you energy and properly nourish your body.

- ✔ **Medium-chain saturated fats:** *Medium-chain saturated fats* are a type of saturated fat that the body easily metabolizes and digests, passing them directly through the liver. This compatibility makes medium-chain saturated fats a great source of energy. They're also high in antioxidants and *lauric acid,* which is a fat that acts as an antibacterial and antiviral. They're abundant in pastured butter, and in coconut products; coconut flakes, coconut milk, and coconut oil are delicious, highly nutritious sources often featured in the dessert recipes in Parts II and III.

Desserts aside, coconut oil is a great fat to cook and fry with because it can withstand high temperatures well without oxidizing and becoming toxic like other fats do.

- ✔ **Monounsaturated fats:** Another healthy fat are monounsaturated fats. Good sources of this fat include beef, green and black olives, olive oil, avocados, lard, and macadamia nuts. Together with long-chain saturated fat and medium-chain triglycerides, monounsaturated fat is a great source of fuel and essential for the body to function optimally.

- ✔ **Polyunsaturated fat (omega-6s and omega-3s):** *Polyunsaturated fat* is another name for the essential fatty acids known as omega-6s and omega-3s. Omega-3 fatty acids occur in nuts and seeds; cold-water fish such as salmon, sardines, herring, mackerel, and cod; and ruminant animals. Omega-6s are naturally present in a wide variety of foods but are also found in excessive amounts in industrialized oils such as canola, soybean, corn, and cottonseed, among others. Omega-6 fatty acids are pro-inflammatory; consuming them in excessive amounts sets the stage for modern inflammatory diseases such as heart disease, diabetes, and cancer.

The body functions best when your diet consists of a 1:1 ratio of omega-6s to omega-3s. This ratio is as high as 25:1 in people that eat a Standard American Diet because processed foods are loaded with omega-6 fats. To ensure you're getting the appropriate omega-6 to omega-3 fatty acid ratio in your diet, get your fatty acids primarily from seafood and other animal sources and avoid processed foods.

Knowing which foods to avoid

The number-one objective of the Paleo lifestyle is to remove toxins from your life while adding back a wide variety of nutrient-rich whole foods, encouraging habits that can improve your health, and lowering your risk of suffering from modern degenerative diseases. Obesity, diabetes, infertility, and heart disease are commonly considered "common" disorders that everyone is at risk for. The truth is that these diseases weren't a common part of humans' evolutionary history for over 2 million years. For example, numerous studies have shown a strong correlation between the occurrence of diabetes, heart disease, and other neurological conditions and the consumption of refined carbohydrates. These chronic inflammatory diseases were reported to be nonexistent in these societies before the people adopted a diet of refined carbohydrates and other industrialized foods. Eliminating the processed foods in the following sections from your diet is therefore vital for maintaining good health.

Cereal grains

Humans didn't start eating grains until the beginning of agriculture around 10,000 to 12,000 years ago. This span seems like a very long time, but it accounts for only about 3 percent of human existence. And as I note earlier in the chapter, our genes and digestive systems haven't changed much since then.

The problem with cereal grains (such as wheat, corn, rice, barley, oats, rye, and millet) is that they all produce compounds intended to keep predators away; unfortunately, those compounds are also toxic to humans. They act as *antinutrients* in the human body, preventing the absorption of nutrients and also damaging the lining of the gut. One such toxin you may be familiar with is gluten.

Gluten is a protein found in wheat, rye, and barley to which a large number of Americans are intolerant. Gluten intolerance takes many forms, but the most severe is *celiac disease*, which causes the body to attack itself, preventing sufferers from absorbing not only the gluten but also important nutrients. Even a lower-grade gluten intolerance can lead to inflammation, which is why grains have no place in a Paleo lifestyle.

Industrial processed and refined oils

Refined vegetable oils and other processed oils aren't naturally occurring fats like butter or lard; they're heavily processed oils promoted as healthy, lowfat alternatives to saturated fat and found in most processed foods. These oils are loaded with pro-inflammatory omega-6 fatty acids and are linked directly to inflammatory conditions such as heart disease, diabetes, asthma, and cancer, just to name a few. Here are the industrialized oils you need to remove from your Paleo diet:

- ✔ Vegetable oils: corn, canola, soy, sunflower, cottonseed, safflower, rice bran, and grapeseed
- ✔ Margarine
- ✔ Peanut oil
- ✔ Sesame oil

Many of these oils are artificial trans fats, the worst type of fat you can consume. They're made by a process called *partial hydrogenation,* in which hydrogen molecules are added to vegetable oil to make it solid at room temperature so it resembles animal fats such as lard and butter. They're promoted as *heart-healthy,* but these industrialized oils are very high in pro-inflammatory omega-6 fatty acids and cause a number of metabolic disturbances. Canola oil, corn oil, cottonseed oil, soybean oil, and margarine are just a few examples.

Refined sugar

Chemically speaking, sugars aren't all the same. Some sugars (such as fructose) occur naturally in foods such as fruits and honey; eaten in moderation from whole-food sources, these sugars are easily digested for most people. Refined white table sugar is composed of glucose and fructose, but in excessive amounts. It and high fructose corn syrup are found in nearly every packaged product, from candy to frozen dinners to canned vegetables, making moderation practically impossible. Fructose is extremely addictive and promotes unintentional overeating. When the majority of your calories come from refined sweeteners as opposed to whole food sources of protein, fats, and carbs, you run a higher risk of gaining weight and developing inflammation, heart disease, and other serious health conditions.

Significantly reducing your consumption of white table sugar and eliminating all artificial sweeteners and highly processed corn syrups from your diet revives your taste buds, allowing you to appreciate the true flavor available in real food. Soon broccoli and carrots will taste like a sweet treat to you!

Soy

Just like whole grains, soy is promoted as a health food, but many soy products are linked to a laundry list of health problems. The problem is that the Standard American Diet contains way too much processed soy, which is directly responsible for a number of serious metabolic and hormonal dysfunctions. For example, processed soy found in most all processed foods causes hormonal imbalances in women and can potentially cause infertility.

A study by the Harvard School of Health back in 2008 revealed that men who consumed the equivalent of one cup of soymilk a day had 50 percent reduced sperm count when compared to men who didn't eat soy. Babies fed exclusively with soy formula rather than breast milk receive an overload of estrogen in their blood — equivalent to five birth control pills per day. Soy also inhibits the body's absorption of vitamins and minerals. These are just a few examples of the harmful effects of soy.

Soy is added to just about every processed and packaged food, sometimes under a sneaky name such as natural flavoring, artificial flavoring, hydrolyzed vegetable protein, hydrolyzed plant protein, or vegetable gum. Keep an eye out for these additives.

Opting for organic, local, in-season Paleo products

Because the Paleo lifestyle focuses on the nutrient density of the foods you consume, buying organically, locally grown and in-season fruits and vegetables guarantees you're eating more nutritious foods. (*Nutrient density* refers to how nutritious a food is relative to its calorie content; high nutrient density means lots of nutrients for relatively few calories.) Research studies confirm that organic produce is higher in vitamins (particularly vitamin C), minerals, and antioxidants and lower in pesticide residues than conventionally grown produce. Antioxidants are what make fruits and vegetables so healthy for humans. The chemical pesticide, herbicide, and fungicide residues found on conventionally grown produce have been shown to be particularly harmful to developing fetuses, babies, and young children.

Organic foods do typically cost more, so if you're stretching your organic grocery budget, focus on the following produce (and a few other items):

- ✔ Leafy greens
- ✔ Berries
- ✔ Apples
- ✔ Peaches
- ✔ Grapes
- ✔ Papayas
- ✔ Nectarines
- ✔ Celery
- ✔ Sweet bell peppers

- ✔ Lettuce
- ✔ Spinach
- ✔ Potatoes
- ✔ Green beans
- ✔ Kale/collard greens
- ✔ Zucchini
- ✔ Squash
- ✔ Hot peppers
- ✔ Baby foods
- ✔ Dairy (full-fat)
- ✔ Beef
- ✔ Chicken
- ✔ Eggs

A few fruits and vegetables are relatively safe to eat when grown conventionally because they're less likely to hold pesticide residues:

- ✔ Avocados
- ✔ Coconuts
- ✔ Pineapples
- ✔ Mangos
- ✔ Kiwis
- ✔ Grapefruit
- ✔ Cantaloupe
- ✔ Cabbage
- ✔ Sweet peas (frozen)
- ✔ Onions
- ✔ Asparagus
- ✔ Eggplant
- ✔ Cauliflower
- ✔ Sweet potatoes

Considering location and season is also important when choosing Paleo foods. Most produce sold in big chain supermarkets is grown hundreds or even thousands of miles away from your neighborhood store shelves. Throughout its long journey to your dinner table, much of the nutrient content is lost. When picked ripe, however, fruits and vegetables contain far more vitamins, minerals, and antioxidants. The best option is therefore to shop at your local farmer's markets, ensuring you're eating produce as close to harvest as possible.

Reaping the Benefits of Eating Paleo

A lot of people discover the Paleo diet because they want to lose weight, improve their health, or determine whether they have some kind of food sensitivity. Others hear about it through success stories of people healing chronic diseases and getting off prescription medication. Regardless of their reasons, almost everyone who tries the diet for at least 30 days feels better and sees improvements in body, mood, and energy level.

The main difference between Paleo and diet plans is that you don't have to count calories; restrict your intake of fat, sodium, and cholesterol; or even starve yourself.

Putting real food first — the nutritious foods your body was designed to eat — the Paleo lifestyle helps you get well and stay well. Reducing chronic inflammation, losing weight, looking younger and more vibrant, and improving your energy level are just a few of the benefits you can expect from living Paleo.

Decreasing inflammation

The human body creates two types of inflammation. *Acute inflammation* is the redness, swelling, aches, pain, and discomfort your body uses as a natural response to heal a physical injury, illness, or infection.

Another kind of inflammation is called *chronic inflammation.* This serious condition often goes undetected for a period of time and attacks your cells, tissue, and blood vessels and can even lead to death. Conditions associated with chronic inflammation include diabetes, heart disease, stroke, cancer, Alzheimer's disease, autoimmune disease, Crohn's disease, arthritis, asthma and allergies, and thyroid dysfunction. These diseases were nonexistent in our Paleolithic ancestors until the birth of agriculture.

Myriad factors contribute to these inflammatory modern conditions, such as excessive stress, sleep deprivation, lack of exercise, and antibiotic use. But the top contributors are the pro-inflammatory foods in the Standard American Diet:

✔ Refined sugars and artificial sweeteners

✔ Industrial seed oils and other hydrogenated trans fats

✔ Refined grains

✔ Conventionally raised meats and dairy products

These pro-inflammatory ingredients are found in the majority of processed foods (breads, pasta, condiments, pastries, and so on) eaten by most people today. Incorporating a nutrient-dense Paleo diet into your life can control, prevent, and even heal chronic inflammation.

Losing weight by improving food quality

Reaching and maintaining your ideal weight is easier with Paleo. The Paleo diet is much more satiating than other diets because of its focus on healthy fats, quality protein, and fiber from fruits and veggies; you can eat less and still feel full. Constantly fighting hunger and starving yourself is a hard life-style to maintain, which is one of the big reasons other diets fail.

Another reason the Paleo diet is so effective for weight loss is that it focuses on the health of your cells and on healing your body from inflammation and other metabolic imbalances. Losing weight is basically a side effect of your improved health. Paleo becomes a healthy cycle: You eat better, so you feel better and have fewer cravings, which makes you want to continue to eat better.

Look younger and more vibrant

Paleo nutrition changes your body's vitality from the inside out. For example, as your body's metabolism and inflammation heal, you begin to notice significan't improvements in your skin, nails, and hair. More specifically, your skin repairs itself from common conditions such as acne, eczema, and psoriasis when you eliminate inflammatory foods and replace them with collagen-rich Paleo foods such as bone broth, gelatin, and connective tissue such as tendons and skin. You increase the elasticity and smoothness of your skin, making it look more vibrant and healthier.

Following the Paleo blueprint also makes your nails stronger and your hair look strong, shiny and thick. Eating high-quality red meat and shellfish supplies your body with zinc and iron, which are essential nutrients for healthy-looking nails and hair.

A lot of people avoid eating egg yolks, but the egg yolk is an extremely good source of biotin, which is also great for hair and nails. (Remember to always check with your doctor first if you're on a yolk-free diet for medical reasons.)

Balanced energy throughout the day

Following the basic Paleo diet plan means boosting your energy levels and having constant, steady energy to function properly throughout the day. This vitality you feel comes from the simple elimination of refined carbohydrates (sugars and grains) and vegetable oils, and other artificial ingredients from your diet and the introduction of healthy fats that boost your metabolism. Coupling these better food choices with some of the Paleo lifestyle choices in the following section — getting physical activity, making sleep a priority — gives you the energy and focus you need to go about your busy day without feeling like you need a mid-afternoon nap.

If you're switching to the Paleo diet from a diet high in processed and packaged foods, your body may take some time to adjust. During this period, you may have sudden dips in energy.

Here are some tips and tricks to help you feel more energized throughout the day:

- ✔ Drink a small cup of tea or coffee.
- ✔ Stimulate your brain with something new. Look up a new word or anything else that interests you.
- ✔ Crank up some music that excites you and makes you want to dance and sing out loud.
- ✔ Stand up, move around, or go for a walk.
- ✔ Get 15 to 20 minutes of sunshine.

Going Beyond Primal Nutrition

As human beings we all have individual differences, but because our genes express themselves in a very similar way, we are all very much alike. Through the course of evolution our biochemistry and physiology have remained similar for thousands of years and that is the main reason why the Paleo template works so well regardless of our individual differences.

The Paleo diet puts real food first as the foundation. But Paleo goes far beyond a diet plan; it's really a lifestyle. Your food choices, movement, habits, thoughts, sleep patterns, and stress levels are all responsible for how you look and feel. This section explores some basic lifestyle strategies you can model to achieve optimal health and wellness.

Managing stress

Being able to manage stress is one of the most important steps you can take toward a healthy lifestyle. Regardless of whether you eat the "perfect" diet or get plenty of exercise, living under chronic stress still puts your body at risk for conditions such as heart attacks, diabetes, and autoimmune disease. Here are just a few of the stress-related symptoms that have a significant effect on your health:

- ✔ Hormonal imbalance
- ✔ Blood sugar spikes
- ✔ Mood swings
- ✔ Food cravings
- ✔ Infertility
- ✔ Fatigue
- ✔ Memory loss
- ✔ Weakened immune system

Managing stress isn't easy, especially in today's busy world. Acknowledging and accepting that you're living with chronic stress is a difficult thing, but developing the courage and strength to admit you need to make a change is important to control this silent killer. I personally struggled to manage stress; for many years, I worked at a job that put me under severe stress, and it took a huge toll on my health and well-being. I knew that eliminating stress completely from my life wasn't possible, but I used some of the following approaches to reduce it:

- ✔ **Learn your limits.** Don't take on more projects than you can handle. Saying *no* to people is completely fine and acceptable.
- ✔ **Choose your company wisely.** Hang around people that cheer you up and stay away from people that drag you down.

 ✔ **Don't dwell on the news.** You don't have hide under a rock, but if current events are getting you down, consider cutting back on news coverage and online news feeds.

 ✔ **Manage your time effectively.** Make a to-do list with the tasks that need to be accomplished the next day, allocating a specific time for each task. On your longer-term schedule, prioritize tasks by order of importance and due date, and either drop unimportant tasks from your list or outsource them to someone else.

 ✔ **Engage in activities that give you pleasure.** For example, walk on the beach, go for a hike, go dancing, hang out with friends, and so on.

Getting a good night's sleep

Achieving optimal health depends on whether you get adequate sleep. Your body just can't attain a healthy state if you don't sleep enough — at least six hours and preferably eight to ten hours. A lot of people ignore this reality because of the large list of things they think they need to accomplish each day, but it must become a priority.

When you get enough sleep, you can improve your tolerance for stress, your energy levels, your mood, and your memory and mental clarity. Your body gets stronger and better able to fight sickness, and you may perform better athletically.

Luckily, following the Paleo lifestyle can help you sleep better for a few reasons:

 ✔ Adding healthy fats and eliminating refined carbohydrates stabilizes your hormones and blood sugar.

 ✔ You have proper *circadian rhythms* (the internal 24-hour cycle that regulates your body's processes). Your cortisol levels are in balance and are highest in the morning and lowest in the evening.

 ✔ Spending time outdoors and in sunlight drives cortisol production.

To ensure you get a quality, restful night's sleep, try these tips:

 ✔ Avoid sweets (including fruits), alcohol, and caffeine in the evening.

 ✔ Eat your dinner at least two hours before bed.

 ✔ Dim the lights and turn off electronics at least an hour before bedtime.

 ✔ Invest in some good blackout shades to darken your bedroom completely.

✔ Go to bed early and rise with the sun.

✔ Make sleep a priority in your life and adjust your schedule so you can get the appropriate amount for your body to rest.

Moving like our ancestors

Another fundamental principle of the Paleo lifestyle is moving like our ancestors, which means engaging in plenty of low-intensity exercise, with some or occasional high-intensity activity. It mimics the lifestyle of Paleolithic folks, who would, say, go for a hunt and then suddenly find themselves running for their lives from a chasing predator. (After all, hunter-gatherers didn't have treadmills.)

In your modern-day life, you can accomplish this kind of movement by simply moving at a slow pace, lifting heavy things, and sprinting sporadically. Slow movement can include anything from walking, hiking, or gardening to performing manual labor. To get the weight and sprinting activity, try lifting weights at a gym and running or doing bicycle sprints; do these high-intensity exercises intensively for short periods of time. Joining a CrossFit gym is a great way to engage in this kind of exercise with the assistance of instructors supporting you and helping you with each step.

Having Your Cake and Eating Paleo, Too!

If you're reading this book, you probably have a sweet tooth. I know I do! Liking sweet foods is part of being human; it's hard-wired into your genes. Eating sweets makes people feel a sense of pleasure and has even been shown to help reduce stress and depression.

But not all sweets are the same. Different sweeteners — honey, maple syrup, refined sugars, high fructose corn syrup, agave — all have a different impact on the body when consumed. I believe that sweet treats can be part of some healthy diet, as long as you know what the limitations are for your own specific health problems and goals.

The recipes in this book are just what you've been looking for to maintain a healthy body while satisfying your natural sweet tooth. Excluding sweets from your vibrant life is unnecessarily restrictive, and restriction isn't what the Paleo blueprint is all about. Your primary goal is always to feed your cells with nutrient-dense whole foods while enjoying living a balanced, sensible life. That is why every recipe in this book was carefully developed with your health and well-being in mind, using the richest, best-quality ingredients packed with vitamins, minerals, and healthy fats.

What you won't find in this book are recipes made with ingredients that weren't part of humans' evolutionary history: grains, gluten, refined white flours, artificial sweeteners, refined sugars, soy, and other chemical-laden foods.

Whether you have a birthday party and need a decadent chocolate cake or you just want to satisfy your natural sweet tooth with a savory chocolate chip cookie, the recipes in this book show you how to make nourishing sweets without sacrificing taste or feeling guilty or deprived.

Chapter 2

The Paleo Kitchen Makeover

*I*n this chapter, I help you completely clear out your kitchen of processed foods and replace them with wholesome, nourishing Paleo foods. I show you how to scrutinize food packaging and read the ingredients list. If you've ever picked out a product at the supermarket by only reading the health claims on the front of the package, you're not alone. Food marketers have done a great job at making a product look and sound good for you with misleading terminology and an organic-looking package. These faulty claims no longer matter to you, though, because this chapter gives you all the knowledge you need to make educated food choices.

I also explain how to purge your kitchen of Paleo no-go foods and replace them with healthier essentials. Plus, I give you an overview of my favorite kitchen tools and appliances to equip your kitchen for making the healthiest Paleo-friendly desserts. Whether you're an experienced cook or just finding your way around the kitchen, my tips and tricks help you along the way. Soon, baking Paleo treats will be easier than ever.

Decoding Food Packages

Every time you leave the grocery store, your mission is to go home with the healthiest and freshest foods possible. However, with thousands of products shouting "lowfat" and "good source of omega-3s" at you, you can easily go off course during your shopping expedition.

Food packaging and labels are essentially the window that allows you to see into the food you're about to consume. But the marketing geniuses behind some brands design these packages with the intention of distracting you from the unhealthy truths hidden in the ingredients list. The key to shopping Paleo is to become a smarter, more educated shopper, ensuring your body gets the maximum nutrition with every food choice.

To begin your understanding of modern food packaging, think of a package as having three different parts:

- ✔ The front of the package
- ✔ The nutrition facts table
- ✔ The ingredients list

Taking the front of the package with a grain of salt

The food companies invest millions of dollars on packaging to convey a healthy message. Take for example the big bold letters spelling out the words breakfast cookies on a box of chocolate chip oatmeal cookies in Figure 2-1. These words, as well as health claims about being lowfat and a good source of fiber, are meant to make you believe these cookies are better for you than a "regular" cookie — even healthy enough to be consumed for breakfast. But are you willing to take the company's word for it? The only way to decide for yourself what will truly give your body proper nutrition is to look at the nutrition facts and ingredients list, which I explain in the following two sections.

Checking out the nutrition facts table

The nutrition facts found on every product is where you find the suggested serving size; the number of calories, fat, carbohydrates, protein, and sugar for each serving of that size; and other nutritional information. It's where consumers have been trained to focus their attention to determine whether a food is healthy. Check out an example of a typical nutrition facts table in Figure 2-2.

The truth is that this table reports only numbers. Reading the nutrition facts to determine whether a food follows your dietary guidelines (such as for diabetics) is important, but it doesn't help you determine whether the product is Paleo. To make this determination, you need to be able to read and understand the most important information listed on a package: the ingredients list (head to the following section).

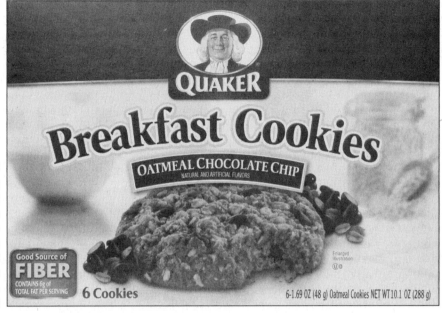

Figure 2-1:
A breakfast chocolate chip oatmeal cookie label meant to look healthy.

Nutrition Facts

Serving Size 1 Rounded Scoop (33g)
Servings Per Container 45

Amount Per Serving

Calories 130		Calories from Fat 20
		% Daily Value*
Total Fat 2g		3%
Saturated Fat 1g		5%
Trans Fat 0g		
Cholestrol 60mg		20%
Sodium 210mg		9%
Total Carbohydrate 4g		1%
Sugars 2g		
Protein 24g		48%

Vitamin A 0%	●	Vitamin C 0%	
Calcium 8%	●	Iron 2%	

Not a Significant Source of Dietary Fiber
*Percent Daily Values are based on a 2,000 calorie diet.

Figure 2-2:
Typical nutrition facts table.

Deciphering the ingredients list

The most powerful tool you have for making healthful food choices at the grocery store is the ingredients list. Unlike the nutrition facts table, which simply displays numbers, the list of ingredients is the number-one way to know what's in your food.

Usually tucked away in small print on the back of the package, the ingredients list is unfortunately often overlooked. Food marketers have done an excellent job designing the fronts of their packages with misleading claims and terminology that make the product sound healthier than it really is. This sleight of hand often distracts people from looking at the most valuable piece of information available on a food package.

For example, consider fat-free and original vanilla ice cream. The fat-free version is certainly packaged to appear healthier, until you compare the ingredients lists. The original vanilla ice cream flavor is made with just five ingredients: milk, cream, sugar, tara gum, and natural flavors. The fat-free version contains a whopping 18 ingredients: skim milk, sugar, corn syrup, poldextrose, maltodextrose, propylene glycol monoesters, mono- and diglycerides, cellulose gum, cream, carob bean gum, guar gum, natural flavors, carrageenan, ice structuring protein, vitamin A palmitate, and annatto. Wow! Do you notice the difference?

Your goal is to overlook any health claims printed on food packaging and understand that foods packed with wholesome, nutrient-rich ingredients are key to optimal health. So here are some ingredients to look for on food labels and avoid in your Paleo lifestyle:

- ✔ Grains, whole grains, and grain flours

- ✔ Refined Sugar

- ✔ Sugar substitutes: sucralose, acesulfame potassium, aspartame, neotame, and saccharin (check out the "Artificial sweeteners: Good or bad?" sidebar later in this chapter for some brand names of common sugar substitutes)

- ✔ Artificial dyes: citrus red #2, blue #1 and blue #2, red #3 and red #40, yellow #5 (tartazine), and yellow #6

- ✔ Caramel coloring

- ✔ Products containing genetically modified organisms (GMO); look for these keywords: soybean oil, soy protein, soy lecithin, vegetable oil, corn oil, high fructose corn syrup, maltodextrin, cornstarch, canola oil, cottonseed oil, and sugar beets

✔ Partially hydrogenated oils, such as vegetable oil and soybean oil

✔ Products containing mono sodium glutamate (MSG); look for these aliases: glutamic acid, glutamate, autolyzed yeast, autolyzed yeast protein, yeast extract, textured protein, monopotassium glutamate, calcium glutamate, monoammonium glutamate, magnesium glutamate, sodium caseinate, hydrolyzed corn, yeast food, carrageen, pectin, natural flavors

Now take another look at the ingredients list for that fat-free ice cream. It has four different types of refined sugars (which definitely don't make this product a healthier choice), and most of those unpronounceable items are food additives, stabilizers, and emulsifiers, which may all be linked to cancer, diabetes, obesity, high blood pressure, and numerous other health conditions.

If you don't recognize an ingredient, your body won't either.

Note: Of course, neither the original nor the fat-free ice cream in this example is a Paleo-friendly version made from grass-fed cream, pastured eggs, and a Paleo-approved sweetener. The idea here is just to illustrate that you have to bypass healthy-sounding claims like "fat-free" and use the ingredients list to determine which foods are the best choices.

Easy tips for determining whether a food is Paleo

After switching to a Paleo lifestyle several years ago, I learned right away that the most important thing I needed to do was to focus on finding foods that contained unprocessed, nourishing ingredients instead of looking at the amount of calories or fat in a food. This shift was challenging in the beginning because I was still learning what real food was.

To make my initial journey easier, I set a number of rules that helped me along the way:

✔ **Buy only foods with a list of ingredients that you recognize and can pronounce.**

✔ **Avoid all products that contain wheat, corn, soy, sugar, vegetable oils, dyes, or artificial or natural flavorings in the ingredients list.**

✔ **Shop for food in the perimeter of the store, where fresh produce and meats are found.** These foods often don't even need a list of ingredients.

✔ **Never stop learning.** Unhealthy ingredients can go by many different names, so keeping tabs on the latest variations empowers you to make better choices.

Defining some of those health claims

Enticing words and phrases used by food manufacturers are often misleading. These claims are approved by the U.S. Food and Drug Administration (FDA) with specific definitions, but you may be surprised at what those meanings actually are. For example, according to the FDA, the word *natural* means that the product doesn't have any synthetic or artificial ingredients added. The problem with this definition is that it doesn't prohibit manufacturers from adding ingredients such as high fructose corn syrup, partially hydrogenated vegetable oil, and other modified food starch, all of which have been repeatedly shown to greatly compromise health. This definition also allows foods grown with artificial hormones, pesticides, antibiotics, chemical fertilizers, and genetic engineering to be called "natural."

Another term to watch out for on food labels is the word *healthy.* According to the FDA guidelines, *healthy* relates only to the numbers listed in the nutritional facts. If the food meets the criteria for total fat, saturated fat, cholesterol, and other nutrients it can be called healthy by FDA standards regardless of the ingredients.

Clearing Your Kitchen of Toxic Foods

Changing your eating habits may seem like the hardest thing you can do, but I promise you it's the best decision you'll ever make. Eating Paleo becomes easier the more you do it, especially because you don't feel deprived of your favorite sweets and treats with the recipes in this book. Knowing that eating quality foods rich in nutrients is nature's prescription for optimal health, you can take this first step with much excitement and rid your kitchen of all the junk.

Eating Paleo is about eating real foods without the huge list of ingredients you can't pronounce. Stick with simple foods and check the labels for suspect ingredients.

Purging the cabinets and pantry

The cabinets and pantry may require the biggest clean-out because many processed foods don't need to go in the fridge or freezer. Get ready to remove those condiments with high fructose corn syrup, boxes of cereal, bags of crackers and chips, and anything else with ingredients you're unsure of.

Here are some more examples of items to discard from your pantry:

- Anything made with white, refined, or whole-wheat flours: breads, pasta, crackers, chips, cookies, and so on
- Breakfast cereals and granolas, granola bars, and oatmeal
- Grains: wheat, barley, rye, oats, spelt, corn, and so on
- Vegetable oils: canola, soybean, grapeseed, sunflower, safflower, corn, and peanut oils
- Foods made with partially hydrogenated vegetable oil and/or partially hydrogenated soybean oil
- Foods with artificial sweeteners and food colorings
- Any condiments, salad dressings, sauces, and other products made with soy
- Candy
- Any products that contain monosodium *glutamate* (a flavor enhancer also known as MSG); look for the following keywords: hydrolyzed, protein-fortified, ultra-pasteurized, fermented, or enzyme modified.

 Although many foods in your kitchen may not fit your lifestyle anymore, your town probably has many people who don't have enough food. As you dig out all those unopened cans of corn, bags of noodles, and other packaged foods, box them up and donate them to your local shelter or food bank.

Tackling the refrigerator

Cleaning up your refrigerator is the most exciting step of your kitchen makeover. You're creating empty shelves and drawers that are wide open and ready to be filled with a diversity of vibrant colors from nutritious foods. You may feel like you're wasting food by throwing away half-full jars and containers, but remember that the benefits of replenishing your refrigerator with real foods are worth it.

The following are some items you want to purge:

- Condiments, salad dressings, and sauces made with refined sugars, soy, or MSG
- Margarine or any other butter substitutes
- Dairy products, if you don't know whether they're made from animals raised in overcrowded farms and given hormones, antibiotics, and feed that's unnatural to their species

✔ Lunchmeats, hot dogs, bacon, and sausages that contain gluten, nitrates, soy, or sweeteners

✔ Sugary fruit juices and other sweetened beverages such as soda or teas

✔ Tofu and any other soy product

Flipping the freezer

The freezer is typically home to convenience foods, which often contain wheat and other non-Paleo ingredients. You may also have frozen meats that don't meet the quality standards of your Paleo lifestyle because they contain sugars, MSG, preservatives (BHT, BHA, and synthetic nitrates), antibiotics and hormones, artificial flavors and colors, corn, soy, canola oil, and wheat. If you can't bear to trash expensive cuts of meat, consider giving them away to neighbors or friends to open up space for organic, pasture-raised meats and poultry and wild-caught seafood.

Clear out your freezer of the following:

✔ Non-organic meats, poultry, pork, and farm-raised seafood

✔ Chicken nuggets, veggie burgers, tofu products, and other frozen snacks

✔ Frozen dinners, waffles, and pizza

✔ Frozen yogurt, ice cream, popsicles, and other frozen fruit bars made with artificial ingredients

Restocking Your Kitchen with Nourishing Foods

When you've cleared your pantry, fridge, and freezer of all fake foods, you're ready to refill your kitchen with real foods —the foods your body was designed to eat. At a quick glance, the foods Paleo recommends on a daily basis are grass-fed meats, wild-caught seafood, leafy greens, and vegetables, fruits, and healthy fats and oils.

Of course, you can also enjoy delicious sweets for dessert. These treats are made with these same nutritious foods, and later in this chapter I show you how to stock your Paleo baking pantry with a just few additional ingredients.

Considering healthy cooking fats

As I note in Chapter 1, not all fats are created equal. Healthy saturated fats nourish every structure and function of the body and were the key ingredient responsible for building big brains in our ancestors over the course of millions of years of human evolution. So which fats should you have in your Paleo kitchen?

- **Butter:** High-quality butter made with milk from grass-fed cows is packed with vitamins A, D, and K and *conjugated linoleic acid* (CLA, a beneficial compound). It's a great, stable fat for cooking or frying at high heat.

- **Ghee:** *Ghee* is also known as *clarified butter,* which is simply butter that is heated to remove the milk proteins (casein). It's a stable fat that doesn't require refrigeration. Look for non-homogenized, grass-fed ghee.

- **Coconut oil:** This miracle oil consists of about 92 percent saturated fat and is known for its extensive list of health benefits. It's a great choice for cooking and frying at high heat.

- **Animal fats:** Bacon fat, duck fat, lard, and *tallow* (beef fat) from grass-fed, pasture-raised animals are temperature-stable fats.

- **Olive oil:** Look for the terms *organic, cold-pressed, extra-virgin, and unfiltered* on the label. Extra-virgin olive oil is a delicious finishing oil to use in salad dressings, and is safe to cook with. Quality extra-virgin olive oil stands up heat well due to its monounsaturated fatty acid and phenolic compounds that act to protect the oil from oxidation.

- **Avocado oil:** Look for the terms *organic* and *cold-pressed* on the label. Avocado oil has a high smoke point, making it a safe oil to cook and sauté with. The oil tastes delicious and is great choice for making sauces and salad dressings.

- **Cold-pressed macadamia nut and walnut oil:** These oils aren't suitable for cooking at high heat, but are safe for sautéing at low heat. They have a distinct buttery, rich flavor perfect for making homemade mayonnaise or drizzling over salads.

Providing Paleo proteins

Protein is essential for supporting your cells, bones, and muscles, and the best source of protein comes from healthy animals. So when buying meat, poultry, and seafood, remember that organic, grass-fed and grass-finished, and pasture-raised land animals and wild-caught seafood are the best options.

They provide you with most beneficial fatty acids and vitamins. The list that follows includes some of the best Paleo proteins:

- ✔ Beef
- ✔ Goat
- ✔ Chicken
- ✔ Eggs
- ✔ Fish and seafood
- ✔ Lamb
- ✔ Pork
- ✔ Organ meats (such as liver, kidney, heart, tongue)
- ✔ Game meats (such as bison, elk, quail, duck, and rabbit)
- ✔ High-quality cured meats made free of preservatives, sugar and artificial ingredients (sausages and deli meats)

Organ meats are nutritional powerhouses containing just about every nutrient needed for optimal health including important vitamins, minerals, healthy fats, and essential amino acids.

To save money on organic meat, poultry, pork, and wild-caught seafood, purchase directly from the farm or fish markets. Check your local farmer's markets, buy in bulk from the farm and split with friends and family, buy from discount stores like Costco or Sam's Club, and buy less-desired cuts of meats and organs.

Perusing Paleo produce

When it comes to fresh fruits and vegetables, you want to look for the freshest produce you can find to maximize the amount of nutrients you're consuming. As I explain in Chapter 1, the best produce is local, organic, and in-season. Because produce doesn't come with an ingredient list, the best way to ensure you're buying organic is by looking for the organic signs in the produce section or by reading the numbers listed on the PLU (price lookup codes) sticker. If the number starts with a *9*, you know the produce was grown organically without chemicals and pesticides. The PLU on conventionally grown produce has a four-digit code starting with a *3* or a *4*.

Here's some nutritious Paleo produce to get you started, categorized by season:

- ✔ **Fall:** Arugula, beets, broccoli, Brussels sprouts, cabbage, carrots, cauliflower, celery, eggplant, garlic, green beans, kale, leeks, lettuce, mushrooms, pumpkins, shallots, sweet potatoes, Swiss chard, apples, cranberries, figs, grapes, limes, melons, pears

- ✔ **Winter:** Beets, bok choy, broccoli, Brussels sprouts, cabbage, carrots, cauliflower, celery, kale, lettuce, mushrooms, squash, sweet potatoes, clementines, grapefruit, kiwi, mandarins, oranges, persimmons, tangerines

- ✔ **Spring:** Artichokes, arugula, asparagus, beets, broccoli, carrots, green onions, onions, lettuce, mushrooms, radishes, snap peas, apricots, cherries, grapefruit, kiwi, oranges, strawberries

- ✔ **Summer:** Beets, broccoli, carrots, chilies, cucumber, eggplant, garlic, green beans, lettuce, mushrooms, shallots, squash, Swiss chard, tomatoes, zucchini. Apples, avocados, blackberries, blueberries, cantaloupe, cherries, figs, grapes, limes, mangoes, melons, oranges, peaches, plums, raspberries, strawberries, watermelons.

Stocking Your Paleo Baking Pantry

Eating Paleo isn't like other diets out there that restrict you from eating your favorite foods just to keep your weight down. Paleo is a lifestyle based on the principles of eating *nutrient-dense* foods, which means your foods pack a lot of nutrients for the amount of calories. So by no means do you have to say good-bye to your family's love for coconut cream pie or ice cream cake. You can continue to enjoy your favorite sweets by simply redefining the nutrient density of their ingredients.

You may think making your favorite dessert tasty without using traditional white flours and sugars isn't possible, but I'm here to show you that it is with a few adjustments in the ingredients you use. The following sections show you how to stock your pantry with Paleo ingredients that turn your special treat into a healthy hybrid.

Eyeing baking essentials

This section gives you an overview of the essential baking items that allow this magical world of healthy desserts to exist. The natural ingredients listed are loaded with nutrients and vitamins and are much different from traditional, refined baking ingredients. Soon you'll never think of making desserts without them. Make sure to always have your Paleo baking pantry stocked with these items:

- Baking soda
- Cacao butter
- Cacao paste
- Cacao *nibs* (pieces of roasted, cracked, and shelled cocoa beans)
- Raw cacao powder
- Coconut butter
- Coconut milk (full-fat from can)
- Coconut oil (unrefined)
- Unsweetened coconut flakes and shredded coconut
- Dark chocolate chips or chunks (dairy- and soy-free, such as the Enjoy Life brand)
- Dark chocolate, 70-percent or darker (soy-free)
- Unsweetened baking chocolate
- Dried fruits, such as apricots, cranberries, dates, mulberries, and raisins
- Grass-fed butter or ghee
- Grass-fed unflavored gelatin (such as the Great Lakes brand)
- Grain-free flours, such as arrowroot powder, blanched almond and other nut flours, coconut flour, flaxseed meal, and tapioca flour
- Nuts, such as almonds, macadamia nuts, hazelnuts, cashews, pecans, pistachios, and walnuts
- Nut butters, such as almond butter, cashew butter, and macadamia nut butter
- Seeds, such as chia seeds, flaxseeds, poppy seeds, and sunflower seeds
- Unsweetened nut milks, such as almond, hazelnut, and so on
- Natural sweeteners, such as coconut sugar, maple syrup, raw honey, and stevia
- Vanilla beans, powder, and extract
- Fats, such as butter, ghee, palm shortening, olive oil, nut and seed oils

The following sections give you more information on some of these staples — fats, sweeteners, and nuts and seeds.

Working with nuts and seeds

Nuts and seeds are a very popular snack for people following a Paleo diet because they taste great and are easy to transport. They also appear in many of the recipes in this book. Nuts and seeds are loaded with essential nutrients and vitamins, but because they're such a handy snack, you should remember to eat them responsibly. For most people following a Paleo diet, where grains and legumes like soy aren't part of your daily caloric intake, a handful of nuts (about 1 ounce) can be enjoyed each day.

Note: Nuts and seeds contain high levels of *phytic acid,* the natural defense mechanism that many plants use to protect themselves from being eaten. Phytic acid is easily digested by herbivores, but to humans it can irritate the gut lining and cause mineral deficiencies in some people. Luckily, studies have shown that the human body can tolerate phytic acid in moderate amounts, in the range of 100 milligrams to 400 milligrams per day. As an example, the phytic acid content per ounce in whole almonds is between 379 milligrams to 466 milligrams.

If you sprout nuts and seeds by soaking them for a few hours, dehydrating them at low temperatures, and then roasting them (like traditional cultures in many regions do), you break down a good amount of the phytic acid present, making them more easily digestible. You can also try blanched nuts, which are easier to digest because most of the phytic acid is present in the skin of the nut. You can find blanched, raw, and sprouted nuts in the bulk section of most health food stores or online at www.amazon.com.

Switching to natural sweeteners

With all the talk and controversy regarding the harmful effects of sugar, a missing fact is often forgotten. Yes, the molecules of glucose, fructose, and sucrose in table sugar and high fructose corn syrup are the same as those found in natural sweeteners like honey, fruits, and starchy vegetables. However, the way your body uses these processed sugars is very different from the way it uses natural ones, and the nutrient density of each sweetener is also much different. So don't believe the saying that "sugar is sugar."

The following are natural, nutrient-dense, Paleo-approved sweeteners that can be part of a healthy diet and are safe to use in dessert recipes. Buy organic whenever possible.

- Raw honey
- Stevia (green leaf or extract) (Steer clear of products that use stevia mixed with other sugars, such as dextrose, xylitol, or erythritol; purchase pure stevia extract instead.)

- ✔ Maple syrup
- ✔ Maple sugar
- ✔ Coconut sugar
- ✔ Molasses
- ✔ Dried fruits

Agave nectar isn't Paleo; it's very high in fructose (higher than high fructose corn syrup). According to numerous recent studies, taxing the liver with this much fructose has detrimental effects on your health.

Using the right fats in baking

Fats are a vital ingredient when making desserts. They tenderize baked goods (creating that perfect texture) and add a special flavor. You want to stay away from all products that contain trans fats and use only high-quality saturated and monosaturated fats. Here are the most common Paleo fats used in desserts:

- ✔ Butter or ghee (organic and grass-fed)
- ✔ Coconut oil (organic, fresh-pressed virgin, and unrefined)
- ✔ Macadamia nut oil (organic and expeller-pressed)
- ✔ Olive oil (organic, cold-pressed, and unfiltered)
- ✔ Palm shortening (made with 100 percent organic expeller pressed palm oil)

Artificial sweeteners: Good or bad?

Artificial sweeteners are a hot topic in the media. The chemical sweeteners are promoted to have zero calories and help you lose weight. However, recent studies have reported that artificial sweeteners may contribute to gut dysbiosis, trigger insulin response in the body and also increase the risk of cancer, heart disease, and even diabetes. Much of this research is inconclusive, and more studies need to be done to determine whether artificial sweeteners are a healthy alternative to natural sweeteners like raw honey. Until then, your best bet is to stay away from using chemically manipulated sugars such as the following:

- ✔ Acesulfame potassium (Sunett, Sweet One)
- ✔ Aspartame (Equal, NutraSweet, AminoSweet, Canderel)
- ✔ Saccharin (Sweet'N Low, Sugar Twin)
- ✔ Bleached stevia: (Truvia, Sun Crystals)
- ✔ Sucralose (Splenda, Sukrana, SucraPlus, Candys)

Equipping Your Kitchen with Essential Tools for Paleo Desserts

Making Paleo desserts is very simple, and when you have the right tools, the task becomes even easier. Most of the equipment you need for making Paleo desserts is the same as what you use to make traditional desserts, so you probably already have many of these items in your kitchen.

Making Paleo desserts is so simple that you really need only four appliances (well, besides the oven, of course). Whether you want to bake a decadent double chocolate brownie or make your favorite Paleo ice cream at home, here are the appliances you'll use most often:

- ✔ **Food processor:** I highly recommend investing in a good food processor; many of the recipes in this book call for one. This handy machine makes chopping nuts, mixing batters, or making coconut or nut butters a quick and easy task. My favorite brand is Magimix.

- ✔ **Handheld or stand electric mixer:** This appliance is perfect for mixing batters or turning coconut milk into a delicious dairy-free coconut whipped cream without wearing out your arms.

- ✔ **High speed blender:** This tool, much like the food processor, is great for chopping, pureeing, and even making dairy-free milk with nuts or unsweetened dried coconut.

- ✔ **Ice cream maker:** You may think you don't need an ice cream machine, but I assure you that after you try the ice cream recipes in Chapter 9, you'll be glad you invested in this affordable device.

Of course, you also need items to prep in and with. The following are my must-have kitchen gadgets and cookware for making Paleo desserts:

- ✔ **Bakeware:** Equip your kitchen with a variety of sizes and shapes of baking pans; I recommend cookie sheets, brownie pans, loaf pans, and cupcake tins.

- ✔ **Cookie scoop:** This handy tool is great for scooping even portions of cookie dough onto your baking sheet. It comes in a variety of sizes, but my favorites are the small and medium cookie scoops.

- ✔ **Cooling rack:** As with any baking, a wire rack allows your Paleo baked goods to cool evenly and quickly.

- ✔ **Fine-mesh strainer and cheesecloth:** These items are great tools for straining the seeds of fruits when preparing jams or for making nut milk.

- ✔ **Measuring cups and spoons:** Baking is a science, so you need to be able to measure the ingredients accurately. Measuring cups and spoons are must-have gadgets.

- ✔ **Mixing bowls:** Ideally, you want to have a variety of sizes of mixing bowls. My favorites are made of stainless steel or glass.

- ✔ **Parchment paper:** Cleaning up your baking pan is a breeze when you line it with parchment paper instead of greasing the pan with oil. Nothing sticks to it!

- ✔ **Wooden spoons, rubber spatula, and whisks:** Stirring, mixing, and whisking batters and scraping the sides of the bowl are easy with these indispensable tools.

Chapter 3

The Nuts and Bolts of Paleo Dessert-Making

*W*hen it comes to preparing meals for the family, figuring out how to fry or sauté isn't hard, and most people can wing it. But things get a little more complicated with baking. Baking is much more than an art; it's actually a science. When striving to give baked goods structure, using the right amounts of flour, sugar, fat, eggs, leavening agent, and salt plays a key role. This precision is especially important when making Paleo sweets, which don't contain gluten.

 Because small differences in the method of preparation and in the ratio of ingredients can significantly affect the texture and taste of Paleo sweets, carefully following the instructions and using the ingredients listed is important. Failing to do so may result in an expensive experiment, and the dessert may even turn out inedible.

So before you begin making Paleo desserts, this chapter gives you an overview of the various Paleo-approved flours, sweeteners, and other ingredients that together give both flavor and structure to a recipe. I also explain how to properly measure ingredients so that you're sure to get satisfying results every time.

Appreciating the Science of Paleo Baking

Recreating conventional desserts and sweet treats without wheat-based flours and refined sugars is sometimes challenging and requires extensive testing to achieve the same texture and flavor. In baking, each ingredient has a specific purpose. For example, flour provides structure; sugar sweetens, tenderizes, and moistens; eggs help bind ingredients; and baking soda and baking powder act as leavening agents.

Paleo baking is also a science that utilizes carefully balanced formulas. Paleo enthusiasts are still exploring this new way of baking, testing to see how ingredients work together and how methods of preparation play a role. The learning curve is steep and has just begun. But today people have a much better understanding of how to adapt conventional recipes for Paleo needs. The main question is how to develop structure and give Paleo baked goods that fluffy, tender, moist, or flaky consistency without adding gluten or grains. Which natural sweeteners will provide that same texture and sweet taste, and which healthy fats should you use to recreate that buttery, rich flavor in your Paleo baked goods? The answers are the basis of much of the rest of this chapter.

Sifting through Your Paleo Flour and Starch Options

When adapting traditional recipes made with wheat- and grain-based flours to use flours that fit the Paleo diet, you may wonder where to start. A number of options are available that, when used in combination, beautifully mimic the structural properties that gluten adds to baked goods. You may be familiar with some of these flours and starches, and some you may have never heard of before. The following sections examine the most commonly used Paleo flours and starches. Which products you choose to use depends on the type of recipe and texture you want to achieve, so I have also included some suggestions to get you started. (***Note:*** When I say "wheat flour," I'm talking about all wheat-based flours, including all-purpose or "white" flour.)

Almond flour

Just like wheat flour is made by grinding wheat grains, nut flours are made by grinding nuts into fine flour. The most commonly used nut flour in Paleo baking is almond flour. Almond flour is lower in carbohydrates than wheat flour and contains no gluten. It's high in protein (containing 6 grams of protein per one-ounce serving) and is a good source of vitamin E, magnesium, phosphorus, potassium and healthy monounsaturated fats.

Almond flour is great for baking cakes, cookies, muffins, and breads. The texture it gives baked goods closely resembles recipes made with all-purpose flour. You can substitute it for wheat flour at a 1:1 ratio. However, almond flour tends to have more moisture than wheat flour, so reducing the amount of liquid and fat and adding a starch or coconut flour can be helpful. Accounting for the moisture difference will help give your Paleo baked goods that same light, soft, and fluffy texture as their conventional cousins.

Almond flour burns more easily than wheat flour. Covering your bread or cake with aluminum foil is a way to keep the tops from burning. This trick allows you to bake until the center is cooked all the way without burning the top.

As a general rule, don't overmix batters or doughs made with almond flour. The flour releases its oils during mixing, and overmixing can make your dessert wet and oily.

When it comes to baking with almond flour, the most important thing to keep in mind is that in order to give baked goods the right consistency, you must use blanched almond flour that has been milled into very fine flour. Blanched almond flour is made from whole almonds that are blanched, have the skins removed, and are then ground into very fine powder. The finer the grind, the better your baked goods will turn out because there's a larger surface area for all ingredients to bind and react with each other. This will assure that whatever you're baking cooks evenly and doesn't sink in the middle, turn out oily and dense, or crumble apart.

A big problem is that brands of almond flour differ greatly in particle size. Brands such as Honeyville (which is what I used in the recipes in this book) and Wellbee's produce a very finely ground almond flour that are perfect for baking. Other brands, such as Bob's Red Mill and the almond flour you can purchase in bulk from grocery stores, don't work well for baking. Their almond flours appear to be finely ground, and the label says they are, but they aren't fine enough for the best baking. Honeyville and Wellbee's almond flours are readily available online.

The best way to store your almond flour is in an airtight container, such as a large glass mason jar, in the freezer or in a cool, dark place like your pantry. If you store it in the freezer, allow it to come to room temperature before using it.

Sometimes the terms *almond flour* and *almond meal* are used interchangeably. Some people refer to almond flour if it's made from blanched almonds and is finely ground, and some people refer to almond meal when the almonds are coarsely ground and made from almonds with the skin on. The majority of cookbooks, chefs, and commercial brands don't differentiate between the two terms, and there are currently no reliable standards for naming the product flour or meal. So the name doesn't really matter as long as the recipe is clear and specifies whether the ingredient should be blanched or unblanched.

Other nut flours

Of course, almonds aren't the only nuts on the block. Other popular nut flours come from cashews, hazelnuts, pecans, walnuts, and chestnuts. These flours are usually more coarsely ground than blanched almond flour and result in denser baked goods. You can use non-almond nut flours interchangeably in recipes, and each nut flour gives the product a different flavor and texture, though for me they don't compare to blanched almond flour for cookies, cakes, and the like.

Particle size greatly influences how successfully you can bake with nut flours. It's very difficult to grind nuts to a fine enough powder at home without a commercial grain miller. But if you're up for the challenge or you don't have access to finely ground nut flours, you can try a few options at home:

✔ Blanch raw nuts before grinding them. Bring water to a boil in a large pan and then let the nuts boil for about 30 seconds. Strain the water and allow them to cool. Slip the skins off with your fingers then place them in a warm oven or dehydrator until dry.

✔ Pulse the nuts in your food processor or coffee grinder and then sift out the larger chunks. You can do the same with store-bought nut flours that you suspect have larger particles in them. If you process the flour too much, though, it will turn into nut butter, so watch it closely and pulse it just enough.

✔ If you suspect your flour is still chunky, you can try adding about ¼ cup of starch such as arrowroot powder or tapioca flour to your recipe for every cup of nut flour.

Coconut flour

Coconut flour is a healthy and delicious alternative to grain and nut flours and makes perfect cakes, muffins, pie crusts, and breads. Coconut flour is gluten-free, low in carbohydrates, and very high in fiber, making it an ideal flour substitute for people with diabetes, celiac disease, or sensitive or allergic to nuts. The flour is made from unsweetened coconut meat that is first dried and defatted then ground into fine flour. The fine white powder has a consistency very similar to wheat flour and is a bit lighter than almond flour. Coconut flour has a mild taste, and when combined with other ingredients in a recipe the coconut flavor is hardly distinguishable.

Because coconut flour is so high in fiber, it behaves differently than any other flour. The flour is very dry and absorbs moisture easily, acting like a sponge. Baking with coconut flour therefore requires a unique wet-dry ingredient ratio compared to other flours. In general, adding more eggs and upping the amount of liquids in a recipe is necessary to achieve the right consistency.

Substituting coconut flour for wheat or almond flour at a 1:1 ratio will not work. If you use this ratio and don't compensate by adding more eggs and liquids, the end product will be dry, crumbly, and won't hold together.

When adapting recipes made with grain flours, substitute ¼ to ½ cup of coconut flour for every 1 cup of wheat flour. It's a good idea to start out by adding ¼ cup (1 ounce) of coconut flour and adding one egg for every ounce of coconut flour used. Doubling the amount of liquid in the original recipe may also be necessary, but it's best to add the same amount the recipe calls for first and then add more as needed. Coconut flour is a very finicky product to work with, and a little goes a long way. If your mixture seems too dry, add more liquid until you get the right consistency. On the other hand, if your batter is too wet, add more coconut flour one teaspoon at a time. On the plus side, you don't need to worry about overmixing your batter when baking with coconut flour like you do with almond flour.

A few brands of coconut flour that I recommend are Let's Do . . . Organic, Tropical Traditions, and Wilderness Family Naturals. The best way to store your coconut flour is in the fridge or freezer, and you don't need to wait for it to come to room temperature before using it. It takes some practice and trial and error to get used to baking with coconut flour, but it's healthy, delicious, and worth the effort.

Seed flours

Seed flours are the end product of grinding seeds like sunflower, pumpkin, flax, and sesame. These are readily available flours that you can purchase from health food stores or make at home. To make these flours at home, you simply grind the raw, unsalted seeds in a coffee grinder or food processor until they resemble fine meal, then sift the flour with a fine mesh strainer to remove any large chunks. Seed flours are a good nut-, coconut-, and gluten-free flour substitute for baking. You can use them in a recipe as the primary flour, as a binder, or even as an egg replacement. Using them along with other types of flours can help add texture, flavor, and bulk to a recipe as well.

The following sections list the most commonly used seed flours in Paleo and gluten-free baking.

Sunflower seed flour

Sunflower seeds are an excellent source of vitamin E, and they're rich in copper, manganese, and vitamin B1. For those looking for a nut-free alternative to almond and coconut flour, sunflower seed flour is a great substitute. You can replace almond flour with sunflower seed flour cup-for-cup. Adding some starch to the recipe helps to give baked goods lightness and fluffiness.

Note: Using sunflower seed flour in recipes that call for baking soda or baking powder causes changes in pH that turn the end product a vivid green color. The food is still safe to eat. This reaction can be a fun and exciting science experiment for kids, but if you just can't stomach green cookies, decrease the amount of baking soda the recipe calls for by half and add twice the amount of an acidic ingredient such as cream of tartar or lemon juice. For instance, if the recipe calls for 1 teaspoon of baking soda, cut it to ½ teaspoon and add 1 teaspoon of cream of tartar. (As I note later in the chapter, baking powder isn't Paleo-approved.)

Flaxseed meal

How do you make the fudgiest, richest, softest, and chewiest brownies without adding any other flour, oil or butter? The secret is by using flaxseed meal. Flaxseed meal is a rich source of fiber, and is low in carbohydrates. It's made by grinding flaxseeds into fine powder and is available as golden or regular flaxseed meal; both have the same flavor and baking properties. It's a great substitute for butter and oil in baking because it replicates that wonderful buttery flavor and texture, and you can use it in place of some or all of the fat called for in recipes. The general substitution ratio for fats such as butter, oil, or shortening in baked goods is 3:1. This means that for every 1 tablespoon of fat, you can substitute 3 tablespoons of flaxseed meal. If you decide to replace all the fat in a recipe, adding liquids such as milk (dairy or nondairy) or water to your recipe is a good idea because the flour is very absorbent.

Using flaxseed meal in combination with nut, seed, or coconut flours helps replicate the flavor and texture of whole-wheat flour.

Store flaxseed meal in the fridge or freezer in an airtight container.

Chia seed flour

Baking with chia seeds is a delicious and fantastic way of adding nutrients to all your favorite recipes. Chia seeds are known for their high vitamin and mineral content. They aid in weight loss, suppress appetite, level blood sugar, and improve energy levels and metabolism.

Chia can be used as the primary flour in recipes or in combination with nut flours. Mixing chia with nut flours creates moist and tender cakes and brownies. Use one part chia flour with three parts nut flour such as almond or cashew flour. It's also great as a binder or as an egg substitute. Adding the seeds to cookies, muffins, and breads gives a nice crunchy texture similar to poppy seeds.

The best way to store chia seed flour is in an airtight container in the refrigerator or in a cool, dark place such as your pantry.

Pumpkin seed flour

You can replace wheat flour with pumpkin flour cup for cup to give baked goods a soft, moist texture. Pumpkin seed flour has a mild, nutty taste and is also a wonderful substitute for almond flour if you need a nut-free recipe. Substitute it cup-for-cup in a recipe that calls for blanched almond flour, and it will give the baked goods a slightly different flavor and color. You can also use pumpkin seed flour in combination with other nut and seed flours, as well as coconut flour and starches.

Baking with pumpkin seed flour adds nutritional value to your recipes, including linoleic acids (omega-6s), B vitamins, fiber, and antioxidants. The flour is low in carbohydrates and high in protein. You can purchase the powder at health food stores or online.

Starches

Using a combination of grain-free flours and starches produces the best Paleo baked goods. Starches are tasteless and odorless complex carbohydrates, and they play a key role in giving gluten- and grain-free baked goods structure, lightness, and tenderness. Different starches have unique properties and behave in different ways during baking. In the following sections, I review the starches most often used in Paleo baking and their specific characteristics.

Arrowroot powder

Arrowroot is an easily digestible starch made from roots of the arrowroot plant. It's often sold as arrowroot powder, arrowroot flour, or arrowroot starch. The white powder has a neutral taste and is very lightweight, similar to cornstarch. In fact, you can sub arrowroot for cornstarch in any recipe at a 1:1 ratio.

Cornstarch is not a Paleo-friendly food because it's derived from a grain that's also most often genetically modified. The powder is highly processed and extracted by utilizing chemicals and high heat.

Arrowroot powder adds to the elasticity and structure of Paleo baked goods when combined with gluten-free flours. The result is a lovely light and fluffy texture with soft, tender crumbs. Adding arrowroot to cookie recipes that call for the standard flour, sugar, butter, and eggs helps create chewy cookies with a more cakey consistency. On the other hand, you can give cookies made with coconut or nut flours a crispier, crunchier texture by adding arrowroot to your recipe, omitting liquids and eggs, and adding sufficient fats. The starch is dry and absorbs moisture during baking, which helps provide that great crunch.

One use for arrowroot powder that I absolutely love is that it gives homemade ice creams the creamiest consistency (which you can find in Chapter 9). When you add it to the ice cream base, it prevents ice crystals from forming, and your homemade ice cream stays creamy and smooth after frozen. It also reduces (or eliminates) the number of eggs you need. My general formula is to add 2 tablespoons of arrowroot powder for every 1½ cups of cream or milk (coconut milk, nut milk, raw dairy milk). You can substitute 1 to 2 eggs for every 2 tablespoons of arrowroot powder.

Tapioca starch/flour

Tapioca starch/flour is a fine white powder extracted from the cassava root. Other names for it include cassava, yucca, aipim, mandioca, and boba. Tapioca is similar to arrowroot in that it improves the texture and elasticity of baked goods when used along with gluten-free flours like coconut and almond flour. During baking, the flour helps by trapping moisture, thickening doughs and batters well. Adding tapioca to cookie recipes creates soft, chewy cookies with slightly crisp crumbs.

Sweetening the Pot: Paleo Sweeteners

Sugar plays an important role in baking. Without it, desserts would not only taste bland but also lack volume, tenderness, texture, and color. Perhaps the most amazing (and scary) property of sugar is the fact that it enhances the flavor of bakery goodies. Sugar is addictive, and most sugars consumed today come from genetically modified crops or from sugar beets and corn and are consumed in their refined form. This scenario leads to weight gain, insulin resistance, diabetes, and numerous other modern chronic diseases.

Many theorize that our Paleolithic ancestors indulged in fruits in season and went out of their ways, climbing tall trees and battling bees, to enjoy a good dose of honey whenever they could find it. Humans clearly have a sweet tooth, and sweet treats have been part of human history. So enjoying sweets on occasion for most people that have a healthy metabolism and weight is okay, and these next sections highlight the best Paleo-approved sweeteners for you to choose from when baking your favorite recipes. Each of the following natural sugar substitutes provides a unique flavor and texture to baked goods and has a distinct nutritional profile.

When you follow the Paleo diet and lifestyle, your taste buds change and become sensitive to sweet foods. A little sweetener added to recipes goes a long way, and you don't need much to satisfy your natural sugar cravings.

Raw honey

The nutrient profiles of raw honey and regular/pasteurized honey are very different. *Raw* honey is the pure honey extracted from beehives, complete with beneficial nutrients and enzymes. The honey is strained through a fine sieve to remove bee parts, pollen, and wax and isn't heated or pasteurized. *Pasteurized* honey is processed under high heat, which destroys the honey's beneficial nutrients and enzymes. Pasteurized honey often has added ingredients like high fructose corn syrup and other sweeteners. Because eating Paleo is all about consuming the most nutritious foods possible, raw honey is what I recommend you sweeten your recipes with. Raw honey has a thick consistency compared to pasteurized honey, which is liquid. Honey adds moisture to baked goods, so using raw honey in the recipes of this book will guarantee you the best results.

Note: Although the healthful enzymes found in raw honey can withstand heating for short periods of time, heating honey above 150 degrees damages it's delicate flora.

Honey is much sweeter than white table sugar. When adapting recipes that call for white sugar, I determine how much honey to use by halving the amount of sugar called for. So if the recipe calls for 1 cup of regular sugar, replacing it with ½ cup of raw honey should be sufficient. I often start by using just ¼ cup of honey in place of 1 cup of white sugar, and then I add more if I feel the recipe needs to be sweeter.

When purchasing raw honey, look for words on the label such as *unheated, unfiltered, unpasteurized,* and *organic raw honey.* Whenever possible, buy local.

Maple syrup

Traditional cultures have consumed maple syrup for centuries; it was first produced by indigenous people living in the northeastern part of the United States. The syrup is extracted by boiling the sap of maple trees, and then it's divided and packaged based on the grade. *Grade A* is lighter in color and milder in flavor. *Grade B* maple syrup is darker in color and has a stronger maple taste. The latter also contains more minerals and is the grade of choice for most Paleo chefs.

When substituting maple sugar for white table sugar in a recipe, I use the same principals for replacing raw honey: If a recipe calls for 1 cup of white sugar, I replace it with about ½ cup of maple syrup. Like honey, maple syrup also adds moisture to baked goods, so when adapting recipes made with wheat flour and refined sugars, either add less liquid to your recipe or increase the amount of nut flour or starch added. When baking with coconut flour, this isn't necessary because coconut flour absorbs a lot of moisture.

When purchasing maple syrup, buy directly from the farmer or look for organic 100-percent-pure maple syrup.

Coconut palm sugar

Coconut palm sugar is made from the sugary sap extracted from the flower buds of coconut palm trees. Immediately after extraction, the sap is boiled down to prevent fermentation until the water evaporates and a thick, sticky brown sugar is left. The sugar is then ground, sifted, and dried to produce the granulated coconut sugar. The product is sold as coconut palm sugar or sometimes as coconut blossom sugar. Don't confuse it with palm sugar, which is a different type of sugar extracted from Palmyra palm trees (or sugar palms).

Coconut palm sugar has a soft caramel flavor, similar to brown sugar, and doesn't leave your recipes tasting like coconut. It dissolves well in liquids and is great for sweetening Paleo cookies, cakes, muffins, and breads. The sugar replaces brown or regular white table sugar cup-for-cup. Like brown sugar, coconut palm sugar gives baked goods a light golden brown tint. The sugar granules are coarser than brown sugar, and pulsing them in a coffee grinder or food processor turns them into fine powder, which is ideal for making chocolates or giving baked goods a lighter texture. When baking with liquids such as water, milk, or juice, you can allow the sugar to dissolve before mixing with the other ingredients. I sometimes use this trick to give baked goods a smoother texture.

Coconut palm sugar is known for being *low glycemic,* meaning it has a slower effect on your blood sugar. It's high in B vitamins and minerals such as potassium, magnesium, zinc, and iron.

Fruits

Fresh or dried fruits are another great way to naturally sweeten Paleo desserts. Ripe bananas and unsweetened applesauce, for example, are very sweet, and they're most likely the only sweetener you'll need to sweeten your recipes after your taste buds adjust to eating low-sugar Paleo foods. These two options also provide structure and can replace binders like eggs. A quarter cup of unsweetened applesauce or mashed banana can replace 1 egg in your recipes.

Dried fruits have concentrated amounts of fruit sugar that can make your recipes very sweet without any other type of sweetener. For example, dried dates, raisins, apricots, plums, mangoes, and figs are all very sweet and add a lovely chewiness to baked goods. You can use one or a combination of dried fruits to sweeten your recipes. You can either chop them into small pieces or blend them in a food processor until creamy and smooth. Then add the creamy paste to any of your favorite recipes to sweeten and bind ingredients.

Stevia

Extracted from the leaves of the plant *Stevia rebaudiana,* stevia is an all-natural sweetener and has been used for more than 1,500 years in South America. It's low on the glycemic index, contains no calories, and is one of the most desirable sweetener for people with blood sugar, blood pressure, or weight problems.

Pure stevia can be 70 to 400 times sweeter than regular white sugar. So if the recipe calls for 1 cup of sugar, replace it with only 1 teaspoon of liquid or powdered stevia. Look for stevia products that have been extracted with only purified water and no other chemicals or alcohols. Be aware of stevia-like products that mix in some kind of sugar base such as dextrose, maltodextrin, xylitol, and erythritol. Some brands of pure stevia extract I recommend are SweetLeaf, KAL Pure Stevia Extract, and Stevita Simply-Stevia.

Baking with Paleo Fats

Fats are imperative for giving baked goods tenderness, moisture, texture, rise, and flavor. In baking, fats such as butter and shortening are classified as *solid fats,* (meaning these fats are solid at room temperature), and oils such as olive or avocado oil are referred to as *liquid fats.* These two types of fats have different properties and behave differently when used for baking, cooking, or frying. Substituting solid for liquid fats or vice versa in baking can be tricky because it affects the texture and flavor of your recipes.

The most frequently used fats in Paleo baking are the following:

- Coconut oil
- Butter and *ghee* (clarified butter)
- Palm shortening (made with 100 percent organic expeller-pressed palm oil; suggested brand by Spectrum)
- Nut oils (almond, walnut, macadamia, hazelnut, and so on)
- Avocado oil
- Olive oil
- Lard

In addition to these fats, other ingredients contribute to the fat content in your recipes: egg yolks, milk, chocolate, nuts, and seeds.

Baked goods made with Paleo fats such as coconut and nut oils turn out nice and moist. These fats also help bind ingredients and contribute to a chewier, cakelike texture in cookies. Coconut oil in particular is the most commonly used fat in Paleo baking because it's highly nutritious and is dairy-free. Virgin, unrefined coconut oil is higher in nutrients compared to the refined version, but it does give baked goods a slight hint of coconut flavor. Refined coconut oil is still a good option if you prefer not to taste or smell the coconut in your recipes. But keep in mind that refined coconut oil has some of its nutrients removed during the refining process. When purchasing refined coconut oil, look for quality expeller-pressed, non-hydrogenated oils that contain no trans fats. My recommended brand is by Tropical Traditions.

Coconut oil is solid at temperatures below 76 degrees. To melt it, place the jar a bowl of hot water for a few minutes.

When adapting recipes, a good rule of thumb for substituting fats is to substitute solid fats for solid fats and liquid fats with liquid fats. Thus, if a recipe calls for vegetable shortening, margarine, or butter, replace it with the same amount of ghee or palm shortening. For liquid fats, swap out vegetable oils such as canola oil for melted coconut, avocado, olive, or a nut oil of your preference. You can use coconut oil in place of butter or palm shortening to make your recipes dairy-free, but please note that the volume and texture of the baked goods will turn out a bit different.

Rise and Bind: Working with Paleo Leaveners and Binders

Although it may seem difficult to give proper rise, structure, and texture to Paleo baked goods, it's not impossible, and there are a number of Paleo-friendly leaveners and binders to help get the job done. Leaveners such as baking soda assist in giving baked goods rise while also creating a light, tender crumb. Binders such as starches and eggs aid in dough-rising while also help to bind ingredients together.

The following section highlights the many Paleo leaveners and binders, as well as some tips and tricks to help you bake perfect Paleo cookies, cakes, muffins, and breads.

Leaveners

Paleo baked goods contain no grains or gluten, so making them rise as much as wheat-based flours during baking is difficult. However, leavening agents do provide a nice rise to recipes made with nut, seed, or coconut flours. Common leavening agents in Paleo baking are baking soda, cream of tartar, eggs, and acidic ingredients such as vinegar and lemon juice. Used by themselves or in combination with each other, they introduce tiny air bubbles into the mixture, making the batter or dough lighter and airier and giving it some rise while baking. Here are four tips and tricks to help you to get the most rise out of your Paleo muffins, cookies, breads, and cake recipes:

✔ Chemically speaking, baking soda is a *base* that forms little air bubbles when mixed with an acid. Therefore, adding baking soda and some kind of acid ingredient such as lemon or lime juice or apple cider or white vinegar to your Paleo recipes will help generate rise. For every 1 teaspoon of baking soda used, add ¼ teaspoon of lime juice, ¼ to ½ teaspoon of lemon juice, or 2 teaspoons of vinegar. For best results, mix the baking soda with the dry ingredients. After you combine the dry and wet mixtures to form the dough or batter, the baking soda will begin reacting with the acid in the recipe.

✔ You get the best rise from baking soda when you use it in the correct proportion with moisture and acid. Acidic ingredients that also provide moisture include coconut milk, chocolate, raw cacao, applesauce, yogurt, buttermilk, and molasses. Typically, you need about 1 cup coconut milk, buttermilk, or yogurt for every ½ teaspoon of baking soda. This combination will give rise and a light texture to your Paleo cakes, muffins, pancakes, and cookies.

✔ Baking powder isn't Paleo because it contains corn or potato starch. A good alternative is to use baking soda along with an acidic ingredient. Baking soda is two to three times more powerful than baking powder, so for 2 teaspoons of baking powder called for in a recipe, I substitute with about 1 teaspoon of baking soda and then adjust for acidic ingredients as explained in the preceding bullet.

You can also make your own baking powder at home by mixing baking soda and cream of tartar. Use 2 parts cream of tartar to 1 part baking soda. In other words, if a recipe calls for 1 tablespoon (3 teaspoons) of baking powder, mix 2 teaspoons cream of tartar with 1 teaspoon baking soda and use this mixture in the recipe.

✔ You can add eggs to your recipes as leavening agents; here are a few suggestions:

- Beat the eggs very well before mixing with the other ingredients. You can also blend the eggs with all the wet ingredients in a blender to create more air bubbles.

- Use equal parts of flour and eggs in your recipes. For instance, if your recipe calls for 4 ounces of almond flour (about 1 cup), add 4 ounces of egg (about two large eggs).

- Beat the egg whites until peaks form, and then gently fold them into the batter or dough. Allow the egg whites to come to room temperature before whipping them. Also, be sure to use fresh eggs because they're more acidic and create more volume while whipping. Adding a pinch of cream of tartar or salt to the egg whites before whipping them also helps give it more volume.

Regardless of which leavening agents and methods you use, bake your product as soon as you're done mixing all the ingredients to get the most rise and the lightest, fluffiest texture out of your Paleo baked goods.

Binders

Binders are what hold baked goods together and provide products like cakes, breads, pancakes, and batter-based baked goods with tender crumbs and a light and airy texture. In the absence of gluten, most Paleo baked goods made with nut or coconut flours depend on eggs to have the proper hold and texture. However, eggs aren't the only option; you can use a number of alternatives for replacing the binding properties of gluten in Paleo baking:

✔ **Flaxseed meal:** Add flaxseed meal to wet ingredients to form a gel. 1 tablespoon of ground flaxseed meal mixed with 3 tablespoons of water or another liquid replaces 1 egg. You can also mix the flaxseed meal with the dry ingredients, and it will act as a binder while baking. Combining the meal with other binders such as chia seeds gives baked goods a nice hold and texture as well.

✔ **Chia seeds:** In place of 1 egg, add 1 tablespoon of ground chia seeds to 3 tablespoons of water (or other liquid) and allow it to form a goopy texture similar to raw eggs before mixing with the other ingredients in your recipe. Alternatively, add between ¼ and ½ teaspoon of chia seed meal to the dry ingredients to help hold everything together while baking. Like flaxseed, chia works well when combined with another binder such as flaxseed meal. Ground chia seeds also work well as a thickener for puddings, jellies, and jams.

When adapting gluten-free recipes for breads or other baked goods that need structure, chia seeds can replace the xanthan or guar gum called for in the recipe for the same amount. Mix the chia with water at a 1:2 ratio and use the thick slurry gel.

✔ **Applesauce, mashed bananas, or plantains:** Bananas or ripe plantains are high in fiber and starch, which gives them great binding ability. You can replace 1 egg with ¼ cup of mashed bananas or ripe plantains. Green plantains give recipes less hold, and you need about ⅓ cup of mashed green plantains to replace 1 egg. Applesauce is also high in fiber and aids in binding ingredients together, providing moisture, acting as a thickening agent, and giving a smooth texture to baked goods. Substitute ⅓ cup of applesauce for each egg in your recipes. Make sure your applesauce is unsweetened; many varieties have added sugar.

✔ **Pumpkin puree:** Pumpkin puree can help hold ingredients together in a recipe. However, it has less binding ability than applesauce or mashed bananas. To replace an egg in your recipes, use ¼ to ⅓ cup of pumpkin puree.

✔ **Coconut oil:** Coconut oil is a really great binder. Adding about ¼ cup of melted coconut oil to your recipes typically replaces 1 egg.

✔ **Puree dried fruits:** Puree dried fruits such as dates or raisins work well for binding and sweetening recipes. They work exceptionally well if you're making a pie crusts or granola bars that don't need baking. The puree is sticky and helps hold the wet and dry ingredients together. Pureeing dried fruits is as easy as blending the fruits in a blender or food processor until creamy.

✔ **Honey:** Honey is sticky, so you can use it as a binder in your recipes. Honey is about twice as sweet as regular white sugar, so be careful not to add too much to your recipe, or you'll make it too sweet. Honey also adds moisture to baked goods, and adding too much may result in a gooey end product.

✔ **Nut and seed butters:** Because nut and seed butters are high in fat and fiber, you can use them as binders without adding too much moisture. Substituting all of the eggs in your recipe for these butters isn't recommended, but you can use them in combination with flax or chia to help hold the ingredients together.

✔ **Starches:** Arrowroot powder makes a great thickening agent for sauces, pie fillings, puddings, jams, and jellies. Unlike cornstarch, you can use it to thicken recipes made with citrus or other acidic ingredients. Arrowroot turns clear as it sets and doesn't make your product turn cloudy. To thicken with arrowroot, mix the powder with liquid until it dissolves before introducing it to a recipe. Your best bet is to add it toward the end or cook it at low heat; overheating destroys its gelling and thickening properties. Tapioca starch is another excellent product for thickening sauces, pie fillings, and puddings. The fine powder thickens sauces quickly at low heat, so you should mix it with cold liquid before adding it to recipes. Like arrowroot, tapioca dissolves and becomes clear, and has a fairly neutral flavor.

✔ **Unflavored gelatin:** Gelatin made from grass-fed animals is not only highly nutritious, but it also works perfectly as a binder and egg substitute in Paleo recipes for custards, puddings, and baked goods such as cakes and muffins. To substitute an egg, dissolve 1 tablespoon of unflavored gelatin powder with 3 tablespoons of water or other liquid. Simply sprinkle the gelatin on top of the liquid and let it sit for 5 minutes to dissolve As a general rule, use 1 ½ teaspoons of gelatin per cup of flour when baking. For best results, don't substitute more than 1 to 2 eggs with gelatin; use another egg replacer in this list. To thicken custards or puddings use about 1¼ to 1½ teaspoons of gelatin for every 1½ cups of milk (dairy or nondairy).

✔ **Agar agar powder:** *Agar agar powder* is made from finely ground seaweed and works similarly to gelatin as a binder. To substitute an egg, dissolve 1 tablespoon of agar agar powder with 3 tablespoons of water or other liquid. Sprinkle the powder over the liquid and let it soak for 5 to 10 minutes to dissolve. To replace an egg white only, dissolve 1 tablespoon of agar agar powder into 1 tablespoon of liquid. Whisk well, and then chill. Whisk again and use.

Measuring Ingredients for Best Results

Using the correct balance of ingredients and precise measurements is essential to give baked goods the proper consistency and density because of the chemical reactions that occur when ingredients are combined and the product is baked. That's why measuring is one of the most important Paleo baking skills.

In this section, I explain how I personally measure ingredients and what equipment I use. I developed all the recipes in this cookbook using my technique, and by following this method, you'll get the best results when making the recipes in this book.

Dry ingredients

When measuring ingredients for baking, precision is key. Adding a pinch more of salt or flour can make a big difference. For instance, coconut flour is very absorbent, and adding just 1 teaspoon more may make your recipe turn out dry and crumbly.

The most common way to measure dry ingredients in baking is by weight or by volume. Personally, I use measuring cups, spoons, and scales. Measuring cups typically come in sets ranging from ¼ to 1 cup and measuring spoons in sets ranging from ⅛ teaspoon to 1 tablespoon. Measuring cups are available as either dry or liquid measuring cups, but I use dry measuring cups to measure both dry and wet ingredients in my recipes. My technique involves the *dip and sweep* method, which simply means I dip the measuring cup or spoon into the bag to collect the dry ingredient and then sweep over the top to level off the measurement.

Follow these steps when measuring Paleo flours and other dry ingredients such as arrowroot powder, cacao powder, coconut sugar, baking soda, salt, spices, and so on:

1. **Dip your measuring cup or spoon into the container and stir the dry ingredient to aerate the product and break up any lumps.**

2. **Scoop the ingredient, overfilling the cup or spoon.**

3. **Sweep over the top of the cup with a knife or your finger to level off the measurement.**

Because measuring the amount of flour in baking is so important, you may want to weigh your ingredients. For reference, 1 cup of blanched almond flour weighs 114 grams, and ¼ cup of coconut flour weighs 29 grams. Keep these amounts in mind when measuring both of these ingredients, and use a scale if possible.

Liquids

To measure liquid ingredients such as water, milk, or juice, most bakers use liquid measuring cups. The difference between dry and liquid measuring cups is that the dry cup has a flat rim and no pouring spout. In all my recipes, I use the dry measuring cups to measure both liquid and dry ingredients. So don't worry about having to purchase a liquid measuring cup; the dry cups will be sufficient to make all the recipes in this cookbook.

Measuring liquids is as easy as filling the measuring cup with the liquid. For more accurate results, set the measuring cup on a flat surface and fill the cup to the top. If you use liquid measuring cups, fill the cup up to the appropriate mark on the cup, and read the measurement at eye level.

To measure small amounts of liquids such as vanilla extract, water, milk, juice, vinegar, and oil, use measuring spoons. Simply fill the spoon with the liquid to the top.

Everything else

Not everything you need to measure in recipes are as straightforward as measuring dry and liquid ingredients. Here are a few guidelines to help you measure proper amounts of ingredients such as bananas, nuts, and chocolate:

- ✔ **Coconut:** Coconut is such a common ingredient in Paleo baking that knowing how to measure it's a good thing. Whenever a recipe asks for a cup or a tablespoon of shredded or flaked coconut, overfill your measuring cup or spoon and then level it off with a knife.

- ✔ **Bananas and other fruits:** When a recipe calls for chopped bananas, chop the banana into small pieces and fill the measuring cup. If the recipe calls for mashed bananas, mash the bananas with a fork and fill the measuring cup with the puree.

- ✔ **Coconut oil:** A recipe should specify whether it's calling for melted or solid coconut oil. If a recipe asks for melted coconut oil, melt the content in the jar by placing the jar in a bowl of hot water. Fill the measuring spoon or cup with the desired amount. If you need solid coconut oil, fill the spoon or cup with excess and then level off the measurement with a knife.

- ✔ **Butter and palm shortening:** Butter is usually packaged and sold in sticks. One solid stick of butter is the same as ½ cup or 8 tablespoons. When measuring softened butter, fill a measuring spoon or cup with the butter, press to release any air from the bottom, and level it off with a knife. Use this same method for measuring palm shortening.

- ✔ **Dry fruits:** If a recipe calls for 1 cup of dry fruits such as dates or apricots, fill the measuring cup with the whole fruit up to the top unless it otherwise specifies that the fruits should be chopped.

✔ **Liquid sweeteners:** To measure honey or another liquid sweetener such as maple syrup, fill the appropriate measuring cup or spoon to the top. Raw honey is solid or very thick, so in this case overfill the cup or spoon and then level it off with a knife.

✔ **Nuts and nut butters:** If a recipe calls for chopped nuts, chop the nuts first and then fill the measuring cup. Otherwise, fill the cup with whole nuts up to the top. If you need to measure nut, seed, or coconut butter, overfill your measuring cup or spoon with the butter and then level it off with a knife.

✔ **Chocolate, cacao butter, or cacao paste:** Use a sharp knife to shave or chop the chocolate or cacao into small pieces and then fill your measuring cup or spoon to the top.

Sticky sweeteners, such as honey or maple syrup, and nut butters stick to the measuring spoon or cup. The trick to getting all of the content from your measuring tool into your mixing bowl is to lightly oil the tool with coconut oil before filling it with the sweetener or nut butter.

Part II
Guilt-Free Paleo Desserts — Time to Get in the Kitchen

Top Five Reasons to Create Paleo Desserts

- Make yummy sweet treats without refined sugar, which can cause a variety of health-related problems.
- Use ingredients that do not include grains, gluten, refined white flours, soy, and other chemical-laden foods.
- Enjoy healthy fats, like butter, coconut oil, and avocado oil.
- Feed your cells with nutrient-dense whole foods while still satisfying your sweet tooth.
- Learn to identify different types of flours and how cutting wheat gluten from your diet can make a world of difference in how you feel.

Visit www.dummies.com/extras/paleodesserts for more great information about Paleo desserts.

In This Part . . .

✔ Dig into a treasure trove of delectable dessert recipes for cakes, cookies, brownies, breads, sweet sauces, and a ton more.

✔ Learn how to make healthy cakes and pies.

✔ Discover how homemade ice cream and other frozen treats can be good for you.

Chapter 4

Brownies, Bars, and Fudge

In This Chapter

▶ Making easy Paleo brownies

▶ Getting behind Paleo dessert bars

▶ Checking out melt-in-your-mouth fudge recipes

*J*ust because you're living Paleo doesn't mean you can't enjoy a rich, fudgy brownie. Paleo isn't a restrictive diet, and satisfying your craving for brownies, fudges, and dessert bars without the guilt (and without all the sugar and other heavily processed ingredients in traditional desserts) is possible with the recipes in this chapter. Using ingredients that our hunter-gatherer ancestors also used, your taste buds will become more refined, such that a little honey here and there is often all you'll need to satisfy that sweet tooth.

I think most people would agree that brownies should be described as chocolaty, moist, fudgy, and chewy. The traditional way of creating such decadence is by using a blend of refined white flours and sugars, butter and vegetable oils, eggs, and cocoa. Store-bought brownies and brownie mixes are far from being healthy and are more like empty calorie treats loaded with artificial ingredients. I've fumbled around in my kitchen to recreate brownies that conform to the Paleo diet but taste as good as — if not better than — the traditional.

If you love a creamy chocolate fudge, I include a few recipes for you to try. These recipes produce a creamy and rich fudge, yet still light and not overly sweet to conform with the Paleo diet. And then there are the fruit bars. This chapter is just packed with sweet goodness.

Lemon Brownies with Coconut Lemon Glaze

Prep time: 15 min • **Cook time:** 20–25 min • **Yield:** 10–12 servings

Ingredients	Directions
Coconut Lemon Glaze (see the following recipe)	**1** Preheat the oven to 350 degrees. In a large bowl, mix the almond flour, arrowroot powder, baking soda, and salt.
2 cups blanched almond flour	
1 tablespoon arrowroot powder	**2** In a separate bowl, whisk the eggs, lemon juice, lemon zest, honey, coconut oil, coconut milk, coconut butter, and vanilla.
½ teaspoon baking soda	
¼ teaspoon salt	**3** Add the dry ingredients into the wet and gently mix with a spoon or spatula to form a batter. Don't overmix.
2 room temperature eggs	
2½ tablespoons lemon juice	**4** Spread the batter across the bottom of an 8-x-8-inch baking pan lined with parchment paper. Make sure the paper covers all four sides of the pan.
1 tablespoon lemon zest	
4 tablespoons raw honey	
¼ cup coconut oil, melted	**5** Bake until a toothpick inserted into the center comes out clean, about 20 to 25 minutes.
⅓ cup full-fat coconut milk	
2 tablespoons coconut butter	**6** Set the pan on a wire rack to cool and then top with the Coconut Lemon Glaze.
1 teaspoon vanilla extract	

Coconut Lemon Glaze

2 tablespoons full-fat coconut milk	**1** In a bowl, whisk together all the ingredients.
2½ teaspoons coconut butter	
½ tablespoon lemon juice	
2 teaspoons lemon zest	
2 teaspoons arrowroot powder	
1 teaspoon raw honey	

Per serving: Calories 271 (From Fat 199); Fat 22g (Saturated 10g); Cholesterol 37mg; Sodium 147mg; Carbohydrate 15g (Dietary Fiber 3g); Protein 7g.

Flourless Fudgy Brownies

Prep time: 10 min • **Cook time:** 15–20 min • **Yield:** 12 servings

Ingredients	Directions
½ cup raw cacao powder	*1* Preheat the oven to 350 degrees. In a bowl, mix the cacao powder, flaxseed meal, baking soda, and salt.
½ cup flaxseed meal	
1 teaspoon baking soda	
½ teaspoon salt	*2* In a separate bowl, whisk the coconut milk, egg, vanilla, honey, and sunflower seed butter.
½ cup full-fat coconut milk	
1 egg	*3* Gently mix the wet and dry ingredients to form a batter and then fold in the chocolate chips. Pour the batter evenly across the bottom of an 8-x-8-inch pan lined with parchment paper or greased with coconut oil.
1 teaspoon vanilla extract	
4 tablespoons raw honey	
1 tablespoon sunflower seed butter	
	4 Bake until a toothpick inserted into the center comes out clean, about 15 to 20 minutes.
¼ cup Paleo-friendly chocolate chips	
	5 Set over a wire rack to cool and then cut into squares.

Tip: You can replace the sunflower seed butter with any nut butter or coconut butter.

Per serving: Calories 130 (From Fat 69); Fat 8g (Saturated 4g); Cholesterol 16mg; Sodium 215mg; Carbohydrate 13g (Dietary Fiber 3g); Protein 3g.

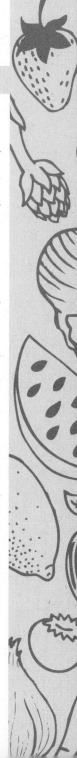

Chocolate-Covered Mint Fudge Brownies

Prep time: 30 min • **Cook time:** 10 min • **Yield:** 10 servings

Ingredients	Directions
¾ **cup blanched almond flour**	*1* Preheat the oven to 350 degrees. Mix the almond flour, coconut sugar, cacao powder, and salt.
½ **cup organic coconut palm sugar**	
⅓ **cup raw cacao powder**	*2* In a separate bowl, whisk the egg, ¼ cup of the coconut oil, the coconut milk, and the vanilla.
⅛ **teaspoon salt**	
1 **room temperature egg**	*3* Using a rubber spatula, gently mix the dry ingredients into the wet to form a batter.
¼ **cup plus 2 tablespoons coconut oil, melted and divided**	
	4 Pour the batter evenly across the bottom of an 8-x-8-inch baking pan lined with parchment paper. Make sure the paper covers all four sides of the pan.
¼ **cup full-fat coconut milk**	
2 **teaspoons vanilla extract**	
1 **cup Paleo-friendly dark chocolate chips**	*5* Bake until a toothpick inserted into the center comes out clean, about 10-18 minutes.
½ **teaspoon mint extract**	*6* Set the pan to cool on a wire rack and then cut brownies into approximately 2-inch squares. Freeze the brownies for about 30 minutes.
	7 Melt the chocolate chips slowly over low heat in a bowl over simmering water (double boiler).
	8 Add the remaining coconut oil and the mint extract to the melted chocolate and mix to combine.
	9 Remove the brownies from the freezer and dip them one by one in the chocolate with a fork so they're covered completely.
	10 Place the coated brownies on a baking sheet lined with parchment paper and refrigerate until the chocolate hardens.

Tip: When buying vanilla extract make sure it is labeled "pure" and avoid the imitation extracts which contain added sugars and are made with synthetic vanilla (from glycoside found in the sapwood of certain conifers or from coal extracts). Products labeled Vanilla Flavoring are a combination of pure vanilla extract and imitation vanilla extract and should also be avoided.

Tip: Make your own vanilla extract at home. Cut 1 whole vanilla bean in half lengthwise, and place into 3/4 cup (180 ml) of vodka, making sure the vanilla bean is completely submerged. Cover tightly and let steep for 8 weeks before using in a cool, dark place.

Per serving: Calories 313 (From Fat 219); Fat 25g (Saturated 15g); Cholesterol 19mg; Sodium 46mg; Carbohydrate 28g (Dietary Fiber 5g); Protein 5g.

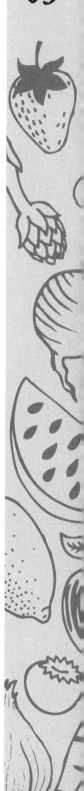

No-bake Chocolate Chip Cookie Dough Brownies

Prep time: 20 min • **Yield:** 12 servings

Ingredients	Directions
Cookie Dough Layer (see the following recipe)	**1** Using a food processor or a blender, grind the pecans into a coarse meal and set it aside in a medium bowl.
⅓ cup raw pecans	
5 Medjool dates, pitted	**2** Pulse the dates in the food processor into a creamy paste.
½ cup blanched almond flour	**3** Using your hands, mix the pecan meal with the almond flour, cacao powder, date paste, vanilla, and coconut oil until all ingredients are combined.
4 tablespoons raw cacao powder	
½ teaspoon vanilla extract	**4** Line a 7-x-5-inch baking pan with parchment paper and spread the mixture until evenly distributed.
½ tablespoon coconut oil, melted	
	5 Spread the Cookie Dough Layer on top of the brownie and use a piece of parchment paper to smooth the top. Refrigerate until the dough is firm, about 1 hour, and cut into 12 pieces.

Cookie Dough Layer

6 tablespoons coconut oil, melted	**1** In a large bowl, whisk the coconut oil, coconut milk, vanilla, and honey.
3 tablespoons full-fat coconut milk	
1½ teaspoons vanilla extract	**2** Add the almond flour and mix just until all ingredients are combined. Don't overmix.
1 tablespoon raw honey	
1½ cups blanched almond flour	**3** Gently fold in the chocolate chips.
½ cup Paleo-friendly chocolate chips	

Per serving Calories 291 (From Fat 208); Fat 23g (Saturated 10g); Cholesterol 0mg; Sodium 10mg; Carbohydrate 19g (Dietary Fiber 4g); Protein 6g.

No-bake Fresh Mint Dark Chocolate Brownies

Prep time: 15 min, plus chilling time • **Yield:** 12 servings

Ingredients	Directions
½ cup fresh mint	**1** Chop the mint in a food processor; add the pecans and pulse until coarsely ground. Place the mixture in a large bowl.
1 cup pecans	
1½ cups Medjool dates (13 to 15 large dates)	
1 cup blanched almond flour	**2** Remove the pits from the dates and process the flesh in a food processor until a creamy paste forms.
½ cup plus 2 tablespoons raw cacao powder, divided	**3** Mix the date paste, almond flour, ½ cup of the cacao powder, a pinch of salt, and the chocolate chips with the mint mixture until all ingredients are combined.
2 pinches of salt	
¼ cup Paleo-friendly dark chocolate chips	**4** Line an 8-x-8-inch baking pan with parchment paper and spread the brownie mixture evenly across the pan. Set aside.
3 tablespoons coconut oil, melted	
1 tablespoon raw honey	**5** Mix the coconut oil, remaining cacao powder, honey, vanilla, and a pinch of salt until well combined.
½ teaspoon vanilla extract	
Handful of cacao nibs	**6** Spread this mixture evenly on top of the brownie and sprinkle with the cacao nibs. Refrigerate until set and then cut into squares. Store leftovers in the refrigerator.

Tip: You can use 1 teaspoon of peppermint extract in place of the fresh mint.

Per serving: Calories 306 (From Fat 194); Fat 22g (Saturated 9g); Cholesterol 23mg; Sodium 23mg; Carbohydrate 29g (Dietary Fiber 7g); Protein 6g.

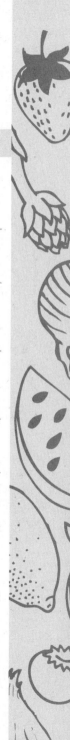

Chocolate-Strawberry Crumble Bars

Prep time: 20 min • **Cook time:** 28 min • **Yield:** 10–12 servings

Ingredients	Directions
2¼ cups blanched almond flour	**1** Preheat the oven to 350 degrees. In a large bowl, mix the almond flour, flaxseed meal, arrowroot powder, coconut sugar, baking soda, and salt.
6 tablespoons flaxseed meal	
⅔ cup arrowroot powder	
½ cup organic coconut palm sugar	**2** In a separate bowl, whisk the coconut oil, coconut milk, and vanilla.
½ teaspoon baking soda	
¼ teaspoon salt	**3** Using your hands, mix the wet and dry ingredients gently to form the dough. (You may want to wear gloves for this process). Don't overmix.
6 tablespoons coconut oil, melted	
3 tablespoons full-fat coconut milk	**4** Reserve ½ cup of dough and press the remaining dough evenly across the bottom of an 8-x-8-inch baking pan lined with parchment paper.
2 teaspoons vanilla extract	
½ cup Paleo-friendly dark chocolate chips	**5** Sprinkle the chocolate chips on top of the crust. Cover the chocolate chips with the sliced strawberries and then drizzle with the lemon juice.
about 20 fresh strawberries, sliced in half	
1 tablespoon fresh lemon juice	**6** To make the crumble topping, mix the sliced almonds with the reserved dough by hand. Scatter the crumbs evenly over the strawberries.
Handful of sliced almonds	
	7 Bake for 18 minutes and then lower the heat to 325 degrees and bake for another 10 minutes until lightly golden.
	8 Set the pan over a wire rack to cool and then cut the bars into squares.

Per serving: Calories 415 (From Fat 268); Fat 30g (Saturated 12g); Cholesterol 0mg; Sodium 136mg; Carbohydrate 37g (Dietary Fiber 7g); Protein 8g.

Chocolate Chip Cookie Dough Granola Bars

Prep time: 10 min, plus chilling time • **Yield:** 5 servings

Ingredients	*Directions*
½ cup raw cashews	*1* Chop the cashews and almonds separately in a food processor and place them in a large bowl.
½ cup raw almonds	
10 large Medjool dates	*2* Remove the pit from the dates and process the flesh in the food processor until a creamy paste forms. You may need to soak the dates in hot water for about 10 minutes to soften them, if you don't have a powerful food processor.
½ cup unsweetened coconut flakes	
1 teaspoon vanilla extract	
3 tablespoons flaxseed meal	*3* Mix the date paste with the chopped nuts and the remaining ingredients by hand until fully combined.
⅓ cup Paleo-friendly chocolate chips	
Pinch of salt	*4* Line the bottom and sides of an 8½-x-4½-inch medium loaf with parchment paper and press the mixture evenly across the bottom of the pan.
	5 Refrigerate for an hour and then cut into approximately five 2-x-4-inch bars.

Per serving: Calories 433 (From Fat 224); Fat 25g (Saturated 10g); Cholesterol 0mg; Sodium 45mg; Carbohydrate 50g (Dietary Fiber 8g); Protein 9g.

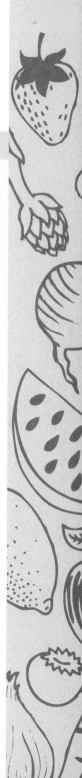

Chocolate Fudge Strawberry Cookie Bars

Prep time: 30 min, plus chilling time • **Yield:** 10 servings

Ingredients	Directions
Chocolate Fudge Layer (see the following recipe)	**1** Using a food processor, grind the pecans into coarse meal and set it aside in a medium bowl.
⅓ **cup raw pecans**	
5 Medjool dates, pitted	**2** Remove the pits from the dates and process the flesh into a creamy paste.
½ **cup blanched almond flour**	
4 tablespoons raw cacao powder	**3** Mix the pecan meal with the almond flour, cacao powder, date paste, vanilla, and coconut oil.
½ **teaspoon vanilla extract**	
½ **tablespoon coconut oil, melted**	**4** Line a 7-x-5-inch baking dish with parchment paper and pat the mixture on the bottom until evenly distributed.
Strawberry Jam	**5** Pour the Chocolate Fudge Layer mixture over the cookie and refrigerate until set.
1 cup fresh strawberries, sliced	
	6 Spread the Strawberry Jam over the fudge.
	7 Refrigerate for a couple of hours and then cut into squares. Top with the fresh strawberries before serving. Store bars in an airtight container in the fridge.

Chocolate Fudge Layer

¼ **cup almond milk**

¼ **cup Paleo-friendly chocolate chips**

2 tablespoons raw cacao powder

2 tablespoons coconut oil, melted

1 teaspoon vanilla extract

1 to 2 tablespoons raw honey

Pinch of salt

½ **cup almond butter**

1 Bring the almond milk to a light boil over medium-heat; remove it from the stove and stir in the chocolate chips until the chocolate is melted.

2 Whisk in the cacao powder, coconut oil, vanilla extract, honey, and salt.

3 Mix in the almond butter until all ingredients are combined. Don't overmix, or the fudge will become oily.

Tip: Check out Chapter 11 for the Strawberry Jam recipe.

Per serving: Calories 258 (From Fat 169); Fat 19g (Saturated 6g); Cholesterol 0mg; Sodium 53mg; Carbohydrate 20g (Dietary Fiber 5g); Protein 6

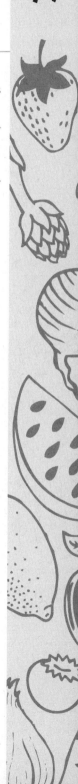

Frozen Blueberry Breakfast Bars

Prep time: 20 min, plus freezing time • **Cook time:** 15–20 min • **Yield:** 10 servings

Ingredients	Directions
Blueberry Topping (see the following recipe)	**1** Preheat the oven to 350 degrees and line an 8-x-8-inch baking pan with parchment paper, making sure the paper covers all four sides of the pan.
½ cup almonds	
1 cup pecans	**2** In a food processor, chop the almonds, pecans, and macadamia nuts until they're coarse ground.
½ cup macadamia nuts	
½ cup coconut flour	**3** Add the coconut flour, arrowroot powder, baking soda, and salt and pulse to combine. Add the coconut oil, coconut milk, honey, and vanilla and process until the ingredients clump together and form the dough.
2 teaspoons arrowroot powder	
1 teaspoon baking soda	
⅛ teaspoon salt	**4** Press the dough evenly on the bottom of the prepared pan and bake until the edges and top start to turn golden brown, about 15 to 20 minutes. Set the pan to cool on a wire rack.
½ cup coconut oil, melted	
2 tablespoons full-fat coconut milk	
2 tablespoons raw honey	**5** Pour the Blueberry Topping evenly over the cooled crust and freeze until firm. Cut into bars and sprinkle the top with blueberries.
1 teaspoon vanilla extract	
Blueberries for garnish	
	6 Allow the bars to sit at room temperature for about 10 minutes before serving. Keep any leftovers frozen.

Blueberry Topping

2 cups frozen blueberries, thawed

⅓ cup chopped bananas

1 tablespoon coconut oil, melted

1 teaspoon fresh lime juice

Cream from one 13.5-ounce can full-fat coconut milk

1 Puree the blueberries, bananas, coconut oil, and lime juice in a food processor.

2 Using a stand mixer or hand mixer, whip the coconut milk cream until fluffy, then use a spoon to fold the blueberry mixture until fully combined.

Note: The cream from a can of coconut milk is what you get when you refrigerate a can of full-fat coconut milk overnight and scoop out what forms at the top of the can, discarding the water. Keeping a can or two of coconut milk in the fridge is always a good idea for when you want to make recipes like this.

Per serving: Calories 342 (From Fat 270); Fat 31 (Saturated 14g); Cholesterol 0mg; Sodium 171mg; Carbohydrate 18g (Dietary Fiber 5g); Protein 4g.

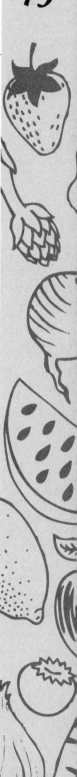

Double Chocolate Espresso Bars

Prep time: 30 min • **Cook time:** 2 hr, 30 min • **Yield:** 12 servings

Ingredients	*Directions*
Chocolate Crust (see the following recipe) **One 13.5-ounce can full-fat coconut milk** **2 tablespoons raw honey**	**1** In a medium saucepan, bring the coconut milk and honey to a light boil over medium heat; simmer uncovered on low for two hours, stirring occasionally, until the coconut milk reduces by half and becomes thicker and darker (similar to sweetened condensed milk).
¼ cup Paleo-friendly chocolate chips, plus more for topping **½ teaspoon ground coffee**	**2** Prepare the Chocolate Crust (see the following recipe), leaving the oven set at 350 degrees after the crust comes out.
Pinch of salt	**3** Take ¾ cup of the warm cooked coconut milk and mix ¼ cup of chocolate chips until melted, then add the coffee, and the salt and stir to combine. Pour this mixture over the crust and bake for 20 minutes.
	4 Remove the pan from the oven and immediately sprinkle the top with the remaining chocolate chips; set over a wire rack to cool. Cut into squares and serve.

Chocolate Crust

½ cup pecans, chopped **1 cup blanched almond flour**	**1** Preheat the oven to 350 degrees. Line an 8-x-8-inch pan with parchment paper, covering all four sides.
4 tablespoons raw cacao powder **1 tablespoon raw honey**	**2** Mix all ingredients in a medium bowl and evenly distribute the mixture across the bottom of the pan.
6 tablespoons coconut oil, melted	**3** Bake for 10 minutes.

Per serving: Calories 260 (From Fat 212); Fat 24g (Saturated 14g); Cholesterol 0mg; Sodium 20mg; Carbohydrate 12g (Dietary Fiber 2g); Protein 4g.

Homemade Blueberry Cereal Bars

Prep time: 10 min, plus freezing time • **Cook time:** 9–11 min • **Yield:** 7 servings

Ingredients	Directions
¾ cup blanched almond flour	**1** In a large bowl, mix the almond flour, 2 tablespoons of the flaxseed meal, and the arrowroot powder, cinnamon, baking soda, and salt.
2 tablespoons flaxseed meal, plus more for garnish	
⅓ cup arrowroot powder	**2** In a separate bowl, whisk the coconut oil, vanilla, honey, and coconut milk.
⅛ teaspoon ground cinnamon	
¼ teaspoon baking soda	**3** Using a rubber spatula mix the wet and dry ingredients to form a dough. Shape the dough into a disk, wrap in plastic wrap, and freeze for about 30 minutes.
Pinch of salt	
2 tablespoons coconut oil, melted	**4** Preheat the oven to 350 degrees. Unwrap and roll the dough with a rolling pin to ¼-inch thickness between two sheets of parchment paper. Remove the top piece of parchment paper and cut the dough into 3-x-2-inch rectangles with a knife, pizza cutter or pastry chopper.
2 teaspoons vanilla extract	
2 tablespoons raw honey	
1 tablespoon full-fat coconut milk	
Sugar-Free Blueberry Butter	**5** Spoon about 2 teaspoons of the Blueberry Butter onto half of each rectangle, leaving a ½-inch border. Carefully lift the empty half and fold over the covered half, pressing the edges to close.
	6 Sprinkle the top with flaxseed meal. Slide the parchment onto a cookie sheet and bake for 9 to 11 minutes, until lightly golden. Set on a wire rack to cool.

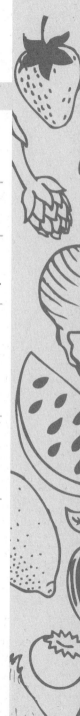

Tip: The recipe for Sugar-Free Blueberry Butter is in Chapter 11.

Vary It!: Fill your bars with your favorite flavor of Paleo-friendly fruit butter, jam, or marmalade. Or for a special chocolate treat, replace the fruit filling with a small square of dark chocolate (70 percent or darker).

Per serving: Calories 137(From Fat 65); Fat 7g (Saturated 1g); Cholesterol 0mg; Sodium 70mg; Carbohydrate 16g (Dietary Fiber 3g); Protein 3g.

Pineapple Coconut Bars with Chocolate Macadamia Nut Crust

Prep time: 20 min • **Cook time:** 20 min • **Yield:** 12 servings

Ingredients	*Directions*
Pineapple Coconut Filling (see the following recipe)	**1** Preheat the oven to 350 degrees. In a large bowl, mix the almond flour and cacao powder. Chop the macadamia nuts in a food processor and add them to the bowl.
½ cup blanched almond flour	
4 tablespoons raw cacao powder	**2** Remove the pits from the dates and process the flesh in the food processor until creamy. Add the date paste, vanilla, and coconut oil to the dry mixture and mix by hand until combined.
⅓ cup macadamia nuts	
5 large Medjool dates (about ½ cup)	
½ teaspoon vanilla extract	**3** Spread the mixture evenly on the bottom of an 8-x-8-inch pan lined with parchment paper. Be sure to use one large piece of paper covering the entire pan and overlapping on all four sides.
1½ teaspoons coconut oil, melted	
⅓ cup unsweetened shredded coconut	**4** Pour the Pineapple Coconut Filling over the crust and sprinkle the top with the shredded coconut.
	5 Bake for about 20 minutes or until the top starts to brown and the pineapple/coconut layer is firm.
	6 Set the pan on a wire rack and allow it to cool; then refrigerate for 2 to 3 hours before cutting into squares. Store leftovers in the refrigerator.

Pineapple Coconut Filling

2 eggs

1 cup chopped fresh pineapple

1 cup unsweetened shredded coconut

1 tablespoon fresh lime juice

1 tablespoon vanilla extract

1 tablespoon raw honey

½ cup blanched almond flour

Pinch of salt

1 In a large bowl, beat the eggs.

2 Mix in the pineapple, shredded coconut, lime juice, vanilla, and honey.

3 Gently mix in the almond flour and salt with a rubber spatula.

Per serving Calories 218 (From Fat 144); Fat 16g (Saturated 8g); Cholesterol 31mg; Sodium 33mg; Carbohydrate 16g (Dietary Fiber 4g); Protein 5g.

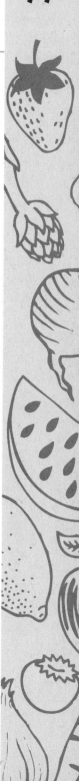

Chocolate Fudge

Prep time: 20 min, plus freezing time • **Cook time:** 10 min • **Yield:** 10 servings

Ingredients	Directions
1¼ cups raw cashews	*1* Line a 5¾-x-3-inch mini loaf pan with parchment paper, making sure the paper covers all four sides of the pan and leaving some excess paper over the edges of the pan.
⅓ cup cacao paste or unsweetened dark chocolate	
¼ cup cacao butter	*2* In a food processor, pulse the cashews for a few minutes until they're creamy.
1 cup full-fat coconut milk	
½ cup organic coconut palm sugar	*3* Melt the cacao paste and cacao butter in a large bowl over simmering water (double boiler).
2 teaspoons organic ground coffee	*4* In a medium saucepan, heat the coconut milk, coconut sugar, ground coffee, and salt over medium heat just until it starts to bubble.
⅛ teaspoon salt	
2 teaspoons vanilla extract	
Raw cacao powder for garnish (optional)	*5* Add the cashew butter, the coconut milk mixture, and the vanilla to the bowl containing the melted cacao mixture and stir to combine.
	6 Pour the mixture into the prepared loaf pan. Tap the pan on the counter gently to remove any bubbles, and then set it on a wire rack to cool. Cover the pan and freeze overnight.
	7 Remove the fudge from the pan by pulling on the sides of the excess paper. Dust the top of the fudge with raw cacao powder (if desired). Wait 5 minutes before serving.

Tip: To measure cacao paste or unsweetened 100 percent dark chocolate, measure it by shaving the chocolate into the measuring cup with a knife. Measure the cacao butter the same way.

Per serving: *Calories 225(From Fat 183); Fat 20g (Saturated 11g); Cholesterol 0mg; Sodium 9mg; Carbohydrate 7g (Dietary Fiber 1g); Protein 4g. analyzed for 10.*

Frozen "Peanut Butter" Chocolate Banana Fudge Bites

Prep time: 15 min, plus freezing time • **Yield:** 16 servings

Ingredients	Directions
1½ ounces 100-percent unsweetened baking chocolate, chopped	*1* Melt the chocolate slowly over low heat in a bowl over simmering water (double boiler).
1 cup bananas	
1 tablespoon raw cacao powder	*2* Meanwhile, add the remaining ingredients to a food processor and process until creamy and smooth.
4 tablespoons sunflower seed butter	*3* When the chocolate is completely melted, remove it from the heat and add it to the banana mixture. Stir until everything is well combined.
1 tablespoon raw honey (optional)	
3 tablespoons full-fat coconut milk	*4* Fill a silicone brownie squares baking mold with the batter. Cover and freeze until set, about 3 to 4 hours.
½ teaspoon vanilla extract	
Pinch of salt	*5* Drizzle the top with the melted dark chocolate (if desired).
Melted Paleo-friendly dark chocolate (optional)	

Note: If you don't have a silicone brownie mold, you can line an 8-x-8-inch pan with parchment paper, pour the fudge mixture evenly on the pan, and then cut the fudge into 16 squares after frozen.

Per serving: Calories 54 (From Fat 39); Fat 4g (Saturated 2g); Cholesterol 0mg; Sodium 23mg; Carbohydrate 4g (Dietary Fiber 1g); Protein 1g.

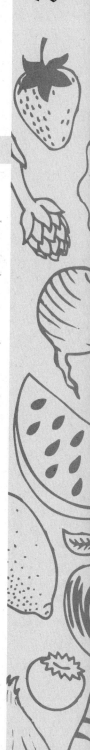

Chocolate Coconut Bark

Prep time: 10 min, plus freezing time • **Yield:** 12 servings

Ingredients	Directions
1 cup coconut oil, melted	*1* In a large bowl, mix the coconut oil, vanilla, and honey, then mix in the shredded coconut.
2 cups shredded unsweetened coconut	
2 teaspoon vanilla extract	*2* Press the mixture evenly across the bottom of an 8-x-8-inch pan lined with parchment paper. Freeze until the mixture hardens.
1 tablespoon raw honey	
1 cup Paleo-friendly chocolate chips or homemade chocolate	*3* Melt the chocolate chips slowly over low heat in a bowl over simmering water (double boiler) and then spread the melted chocolate evenly over the top of the frozen coconut.
	4 Return the pan to the freezer and, after the chocolate has set, chop the bark into small pieces. Keep frozen.

Tip: You can find a recipe for homemade chocolate in Chapter 7.

Per serving: Calories 376 (From Fat 304); Fat 35g (Saturated 28g); Cholesterol 0mg; Sodium 5mg; Carbohydrate 17g (Dietary Fiber 3g); Protein 2g.

Chocolate Chunk Macadamia Nut Fudge

Prep time: 15 min, plus freezing time • **Yield:** 8 servings

Ingredients	Directions
1 cup raw macadamia nuts ⅓ cup almond milk 2 teaspoons vanilla extract 1 tablespoon coconut oil, melted 1 tablespoon raw honey Pinch of salt 1 tablespoon cacao butter ⅓ cup Paleo-friendly chocolate chunks	**1** Place the macadamia nuts, almond milk, vanilla, coconut oil, honey, and salt in a food processor or high-speed blender and process until creamy and smooth. **2** Melt the cacao butter slowly in a bowl over simmering water (double boiler). **3** Remove the cacao butter from the stove and using a rubber spatula mix in the macadamia nut mixture; fold in the chocolate chunks. **4** Spread mixture evenly across the bottom of a 7-x-5-inch baking dish lined with parchment paper. **5** Freeze until hardened and then cut into squares. Keep leftovers frozen.

Per serving: Calories 216 (From Fat 175); Fat 20g (Saturated 7g); Cholesterol 0mg; Sodium 25mg; Carbohydrate 11g (Dietary Fiber 8g); Protein 2g.

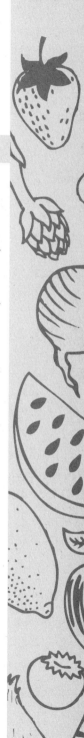

Chapter 5

Classic Breads

In This Chapter

▶ Finding alternatives to wheat and grain flours

▶ Baking a variety of quick breads

Transitioning to Paleo is very difficult for some people because they're so used to eating bread. Cutting out bread completely in the beginning is so hard that most people aren't willing to do it. I get it: Who doesn't love a piece of soft, warm, freshly baked dessert bread smothered with butter? Luckily, you can make Paleo-approved breads by swapping nut and coconut flours, as well as starchy tubers such as tapioca and arrowroot flours.

To ensure the breads turn out light and fluffy and don't sink in the middle, make sure to use blanched almond flour that has been ground very finely. If you're unsure whether your flour is fine enough, use a strainer to sift out larger chunks and/or pulse the flour in your food processor a few times.

Some of the bread recipes you find in this chapter are baked using other unique ingredients. One example is the Avocado Chocolate Bread. Baking breads with avocados adds healthy fats as well as a wonderful texture. And because the flavor of avocados is so mild, you don't taste it all!

If your idea of dessert is more along the lines of a regular piece of toast with some nut butter or jam, I've also included a recipe for Paleo Sandwich Bread in this chapter. (Of course, you can also use it for mealtime sandwiches.) Many people have told me this bread is just what they've been looking for and really resembles sandwich bread.

Paleo Sandwich Bread

Prep time: 15 min • **Cook time:** 35 min • **Yield:** 10 servings

Ingredients	*Directions*
2 cups blanched almond flour	*1* Preheat the oven to 350 degrees. In a large bowl, mix the almond flour, flaxseed meal, flaxseeds, salt, baking soda, and arrowroot powder.
⅓ cup plus 1 tablespoon flaxseed meal	
1 teaspoon whole flaxseeds, plus more for garnish (optional)	*2* In a saucepan, melt the butter over medium heat and let cool for 5 minutes. Whisk the melted butter with the eggs, vinegar, and yogurt.
½ teaspoon salt	
1 teaspoon baking soda	*3* Using a rubber spatula, gently mix the wet and dry ingredients to form a batter; don't overmix, or the batter will get oily and dense.
½ cup arrowroot powder	
6 tablespoons pastured butter	*4* Pour the batter into an 8½-x-4½-inch medium loaf pan lined with parchment paper. Sprinkle the top with whole flaxseeds (if desired).
4 eggs	
1 teaspoon apple cider vinegar	*5* Bake until a toothpick inserted into the center of the bread comes out clean, about 35 minutes.
½ cup plain Greek yogurt	
	6 Let bread cool on a wire rack; cut into thin slices and serve. To preserve freshness, wrap the bread in paper towel, place it inside a zip-top bag or airtight container, and store it in the refrigerator for about 1 week.

Tip: To help give your bread rise, you can separate the eggs and, using an electric mixer, beat the egg whites with a pinch of cream of tartar until they form stiff peaks. Then gently fold this mixture into your batter as the last step.

Vary It! You can use coconut cream in place of the Greek yogurt. It's the thick cream that forms at the top of a can of full-fat coconut milk when you leave it in the fridge for more than 12 hours.

Per serving: *Calories 280 (From Fat 201); Fat 22g (Saturated 7g); Cholesterol 94mg; Sodium 282mg; Carbohydrate 13g (Dietary Fiber 4g); Protein 9g.*

Best Chocolate Zucchini Bread

Prep time: 20 min • **Cook time:** 35 min • **Yield:** 10 servings

Ingredients	Directions
1½ cups blanched almond flour	**1** Preheat the oven to 350 degrees. In a bowl, mix the almond flour, baking soda, cacao powder, cinnamon, and salt.
1½ teaspoons baking soda	
¼ cup raw cacao powder	
2 teaspoons ground cinnamon	**2** In a separate bowl, beat the egg and then add the yogurt, coconut oil, vanilla, honey, and vinegar. Mix until well combined.
¼ teaspoon salt	
1 large room temperature egg	**3** Stir the zucchini, pecans, and chocolate chips into the wet mixture.
¼ cup plain Greek yogurt	
¼ cup coconut oil, melted	**4** Using a rubber spatula, gently mix the wet and dry ingredients together. Don't overmix.
1 teaspoon vanilla extract	
3 tablespoons raw honey	**5** Spoon the batter into an 8½-x-4½-inch medium loaf pan lined with parchment paper. Bake until a toothpick inserted into the center comes out clean, about 35 minutes.
1 teaspoon apple cider vinegar	
1 cup finely grated zucchini	
½ cup pecans, chopped	**6** Cool on a wire rack. Store in an airtight container in the refrigerator for about 1 week.
½ cup Paleo-friendly chocolate chips	

Per serving: Calories 290 (From Fat 203); Fat 23g (Saturated 9g); Cholesterol 19mg; Sodium 265mg; Carbohydrate 19g (Dietary Fiber 4g); Protein 7g.

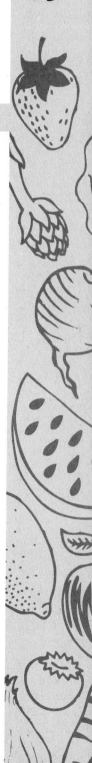

Avocado Chocolate Bread

Prep time: 20 min • **Cook time:** 45 min • **Yield:** 10 servings

Ingredients	Directions

Ingredients

1½ cups mashed avocado
(about 2 small avocados)

3 tablespoons coconut oil,
melted

1 teaspoon vanilla extract

2½ tablespoons coconut
cream

3 tablespoons raw honey

2 eggs

½ cup pecans, chopped

2 cups blanched
almond flour

1 teaspoon baking soda

¼ cup raw cacao powder

½ teaspoon salt

⅓ cup Paleo-friendly
chocolate chips, plus more
for garnish

Directions

1 Preheat the oven to 350 degrees. Pulse the avocado in a food processor until creamy.

2 Add the coconut oil, vanilla, coconut cream, honey, and eggs and pulse to combine.

3 In a large bowl, mix the pecans, almond flour, baking soda, cacao powder, salt, and chocolate chips.

4 Combine the wet and dry ingredients and mix gently with a rubber spatula. Don't overmix.

5 Spoon the batter into an 8½-x-4½-inch medium loaf pan lined with parchment paper, spreading it across the pan with a spatula. Sprinkle the top with chocolate chips.

6 Bake until a toothpick inserted into the center of the bread comes out clean, about 45 minutes.

7 Let it cool on a wire rack. To preserve freshness, place inside an airtight container and store in the refrigerator for about 1 week.

Note: The cream from a can of coconut milk is what you get when you refrigerate a can of full-fat coconut milk for more than 12 hours and scoop out what forms at the top of the can, discarding the water.

Tip: I recommend you use Hass avocados to make this recipe because they aren't bitter like other types of avocados, which may give a bitter aftertaste to this bread.

Per serving: Calories 342 (From Fat 243); Fat 27g (Saturated 8g); Cholesterol 0mg; Sodium 269mg; Carbohydrate 21g (Dietary Fiber 6g); Protein 8g.

Black Bottom Banana Bread

Prep time: 15 min • **Cook time:** 50 min • **Yield:** 10 servings

Ingredients	Directions
1½ cups blanched almond flour	**1** Preheat the oven to 350 degrees. In a medium bowl, mix the almond flour, baking soda, and salt.
1½ teaspoons baking soda	
½ teaspoon salt	**2** Pulse the banana, coconut oil, vanilla, egg, and honey in a food processor until combined.
1½ cups chopped banana	
4 tablespoons coconut oil, melted	**3** Mix the wet and dry ingredients to form a batter. Don't overmix, or the batter will become oily anddense.
1 teaspoon vanilla extract	
1 large room temperature egg	**4** Divide the batter in half. Add the cacao powder and chocolate chips to one half and pour it into the bottom of an 8½-x-4½-inch medium loaf pan lined with parchment paper.
1 tablespoon raw honey	
¼ cup raw cacao powder	
¼ cup Paleo-friendly chocolate chips	**5** Spoon the other half of the batter on top and bake until a toothpick inserted into the center comes out clean, about 50 minutes. Cover the pan with aluminum foil after 30 minutes of baking to prevent the top from overbrowning.

Tip: Apple bananas enhance the flavor of this bread, so consider using them if you can find them at your local stores or online. Apple bananas are smaller than the more common varieties and have a distinct sweet yet tangy flavor. As they ripen, they become sweeter and develop a unique tropical flavor resembling a blend of pineapple and strawberries. They grow year round in tropical regions and are readily available in Hawaii, Honduras, Malaysia, and Mexico.

Per serving: Calories 223(From Fat 152); Fat 17g (Saturated 7g); Cholesterol 19mg; Sodium 319mg; Carbohydrate 15g (Dietary Fiber 3g); Protein 6g.

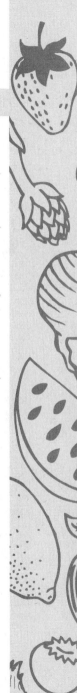

Blueberry Bread with Lemon Glaze

Prep time: 20 min • **Cook time:** 40 min • **Yield:** 10 servings

Ingredients	Directions
2 cups blanched almond flour	*1* Preheat the oven to 350 degrees. In a large bowl, mix the almond flour, baking soda, and salt.
1 teaspoon baking soda	
½ teaspoon salt	*2* In a separate bowl, whisk the coconut milk, eggs, 3 tablespoons of the honey, the vanilla, coconut oil, and lemon zest; then stir in the fresh blueberries.
¼ cup full-fat coconut milk	
2 room temperature eggs	*3* Gently mix the wet and dry ingredients to form a batter; don't overmix, or the batter will get oily and dense.
3 tablespoons plus ¼ teaspoon raw honey, divided	
2 teaspoons vanilla extract	*4* Spoon the batter into an 8½-x-4½-inch medium loaf pan lined with parchment paper.
½ cup coconut oil, melted	
2 teaspoons lemon zest	*5* Bake until a toothpick inserted into the center comes out clean, about 40 to 45 minutes. Meanwhile, whisk the lemon juice with the remaining honey to make the glaze.
¾ cup fresh blueberries	
½ tablespoon fresh lemon juice	*6* Poke a few small holes across the top of the bread with a toothpick and brush on the glaze.
	7 Set the pan over a wire rack to cool. To preserve freshness, place inside an airtight container and store in the refrigerator for about 1 week.

Per serving: Calories 276 (From Fat 214); Fat 24g (Saturated 12g); Cholesterol 37mg; Sodium 266mg; Carbohydrate 12g (Dietary Fiber 3g); Protein 6g.

Chocolate Chip Bread

Prep time: 20 min • **Cook time:** 45 min • **Yield:** 10 servings

Ingredients	*Directions*
Chocolate Glaze (see the following recipe)	**1** Preheat the oven to 350 degrees. Mix the almond flour, arrowroot powder, baking soda, and salt.
2 cups blanched almond flour	
1 tablespoon arrowroot powder	**2** In a separate bowl, whisk the eggs, butter, coconut milk, honey, vinegar, and vanilla.
½ teaspoon baking soda	
¼ teaspoon salt	**3** Add the wet ingredients to the dry ingredients and gently mix with a rubber spatula until just combined. Don't overmix.
2 room temperature eggs	
6 tablespoons pastured butter, softened	**4** Pour the batter into an 8½-x-4½-inch medium loaf pan lined with parchment paper. Make sure the paper covers all four sides of the pan.
⅓ cup full-fat coconut milk	
3 tablespoons raw honey	**5** Bake until a toothpick inserted into the center comes out clean, about 45 minutes. Set the pan on a wire rack to cool.
2 teaspoons apple cider vinegar	
1 teaspoon vanilla extract	**6** Pour the Chocolate Glaze over the top of the cooled bread and allow the chocolate to set for a few minutes before removing the bread from the pan. To preserve freshness, place inside an airtight container and store in the refrigerator for about 2 week.
½ cup Paleo-friendly dark chocolate chips	

Chocolate Glaze

⅓ cup Paleo-friendly dark chocolate chips	**1** Slowly melt the chocolate over low heat in a bowl over simmering water (double boiler).
2 tablespoons full-fat coconut milk	**2** Stir the coconut milk into the melted chocolate until everything is combined and smooth.

Per serving: Calories 339 (From Fat 261); Fat 29g (Saturated 13g); Cholesterol 55mg; Sodium 145mg; Carbohydrate 22g (Dietary Fiber 5g); Protein 8g.

Marble Bread

Prep time: 25 min • **Cook time:** 30 min • **Yield:** 10 servings

Ingredients	*Directions*
1½ cups blanched almond flour	**1** Preheat the oven to 350 degrees. In a medium bowl, mix the almond flour, baking soda, and salt.
1 teaspoon baking soda	
½ teaspoon salt	**2** In a separate bowl, beat the butter and coconut sugar with an electric mixer until fluffy. Add the eggs one at a time, beating after each addition, and then mix in the coconut milk and vanilla until smooth.
4 tablespoons room temperature pastured butter	
¼ cup organic coconut palm sugar	**3** Using a rubber spatula, gently mix the almond flour mixture into the wet ingredients. Gently fold in ⅓ cup of the macadamia nuts (if desired), reserving the rest to garnish the top of the bread.
2 large eggs	
½ cup full-fat coconut milk	
2 teaspoons vanilla extract	**4** Remove about ½ cup of the batter and place it in a separate bowl. Add the cacao powder to this batter and mix to combine.
¼ to ½ cup chopped macadamia nuts (optional)	
1½ tablespoons raw cacao powder	**5** Line an 8½-x-4½-inch medium loaf pan with parchment paper and pour in half the vanilla batter, evenly coating the bottom of the pan. Then pour in the chocolate batter and top it off with the remaining vanilla batter.
¼ cup Paleo-friendly chocolate chips for garnish (optional)	
	6 Use a knife to swirl the chocolate and vanilla batters together in the pan. Sprinkle the reserved macadamia nuts and chocolate chips on top (if desired).
	7 Bake until a toothpick inserted into the center of the bread comes out clean, about 30 minutes.
	8 Cool on a wire rack completely before serving. To preserve freshness, place inside an airtight container and store in the refrigerator for about 2 week.

Per serving: Calories 202 (From Fat 148); Fat 17g (Saturated 7g); Cholesterol 50mg; Sodium 267mg; Carbohydrate 11g (Dietary Fiber 2g); Protein 5g.

Chocolate Chip Banana Bread

Prep time: 20 min • **Cook time:** 45–50 min • **Yield:** 10 servings

Ingredients	*Directions*
1½ cups chopped banana	*1* Preheat the oven to 350 degrees. Pulse the bananas, eggs, vanilla, honey, and coconut oil in a food processor. Add the pecans and pulse to break them into small pieces.
3 eggs	
1 tablespoon vanilla extract	
1 tablespoon raw honey	*2* In a large bowl, mix the almond flour, baking soda, and salt.
¼ cup coconut oil, melted	
1 cup whole raw pecans	*3* Using a rubber spatula, gently mix the dry and wet ingredients together. Fold in the chocolate chips.
2 cups blanched almond flour	
1 teaspoon baking soda	*4* Pour the batter into an 8½-x-4½-inch medium loaf pan lined with parchment paper. Make sure the paper covers all four sides of the pan.
½ teaspoon salt	
⅓ cup Paleo-friendly chocolate chips	*5* Bake until a toothpick inserted into the center of the bread comes out clean, about 45 to 50 minutes.
	6 Allow the pan to cool on a wire rack. To preserve freshness, place inside an airtight container and store in the refrigerator for 1 to 2 weeks.

Tip: Apple bananas enhance the flavor of this bread, so consider using them if you can find them at your local stores or online.

Per serving: Calories 337 (From Fat 249); Fat 28g (Saturated 8g); Cholesterol 56mg; Sodium 272mg; Carbohydrate 18g (Dietary Fiber 5g); Protein 8g.

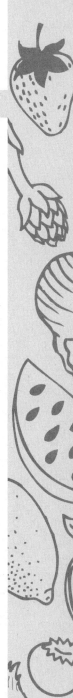

Avocado Banana Bread

Prep time: 20 min • **Cook time:** 45–50 min • **Yield:** 10 servings

Ingredients	Directions
1½ cups blanched almond flour	**1** Preheat the oven to 350 degrees. In a large bowl, mix the almond flour, baking soda, and salt.
1½ teaspoons baking soda	
½ teaspoon salt	**2** Pulse the avocado and bananas in a food processor until creamy. Add the coconut oil, vanilla, honey, and egg, and pulse to combine.
¾ cup mashed avocado	
¾ cup chopped banana	**3** Using a rubber spatula gently mix the wet ingredients into the dry ingredients and mix to form a batter.
3 tablespoons coconut oil, melted	
1 teaspoon vanilla extract	**4** Line an 8½-x-4½-inch medium loaf pan with parchment paper and spread the batter across the pan.
3 tablespoons raw honey	
1 large room temperature egg	**5** Bake until a toothpick inserted into the center comes out clean, about 45 to 50 minutes. To preserve freshness, place inside an airtight container and store in the refrigerator for about 1 week.
⅓ cup macadamia nuts, chopped	

Tip: I recommend you use Hass avocados to make this recipe. Other types of avocados may give this bread a bitter aftertaste.

Tip: Apple bananas enhance the flavor of this bread, so consider using them if you can find them at your local stores or online.

Per serving: Calories 218 (From Fat 160); Fat 18g (Saturated 5g); Cholesterol 19mg; Sodium 320mg; Carbohydrate 13g (Dietary Fiber 3g); Protein 5g.

Chapter 6

Cakes and Pies

In This Chapter

▶ Celebrating special occasions with yummy Paleo cakes

▶ Creating luscious, easy Paleo pies

Celebrating special occasions with a piece of cake or pie is traditionally engrained in Western culture. Imagine ending a child's birthday party without a mouth-watering cake brimming with candles, or sitting down to Thanksgiving dinner with no pumpkin pie. It would be no fun.

Paleo isn't like other diet programs that leave you feeling like the only person at the party who can't enjoy a piece of cake. When you follow a Paleo lifestyle, you can commemorate special events with sweets, too.

In this chapter, I show you how you can prepare cakes and pies, using healthful and wholesome ingredients. This way, when an occasion arises, you can easily make something to share and celebrate with everyone at the party. No one will notice the difference in taste (or presentation) between your Paleo cake or pie and traditional ones made with traditional ingredients.

I start this chapter off with a simple recipe for a decadent chocolate cake. It's light, fluffy, moist, chocolaty, and not overly sweet. The middle layer is even made out of a creamy, dairy-free chocolate ganache, so you don't feel like you're following any kind of special diet.

Note: Many of the recipes in this chapter call for greasing a pan with coconut oil; that oil is in addition to any coconut oil that may be in the ingredients lists for those recipes.

Chocolate Cake

Prep time: 25 min • **Cook time:** 2 hr, 50 min **Yield:** 10 servings

Ingredients	Directions
Chocolate Ganache (see the following recipe) (prepare in advance)	*1* Preheat the oven to 350 degrees. Grease the bottom and sides of a 7-inch springform pan with coconut oil and line the bottom with parchment paper.
Chocolate Frosting (see the following recipe)	
3 cups blanched almond flour	*2* In a large bowl, mix the almond flour, coconut flour, cacao powder, coconut sugar, baking soda, and salt.
¼ cup coconut flour	
¾ cup raw cacao powder	*3* In a separate bowl, whisk the coconut oil, coconut milk, eggs, vanilla, and honey.
½ cup organic coconut palm sugar	
2 teaspoons baking soda	*4* Using a rubber spatula, gently mix the dry ingredients and wet ingredients together. Don't overmix.
1 teaspoon salt	
½ cup coconut oil, melted	*5* Pour the batter into the prepared pan and bake until a toothpick inserted into the center comes out clean, approximately 45 to 50 minutes. (If it needs more time, cover the cake with aluminum foil and lower the heat to 325 degrees.)
1 cup full-fat coconut milk	
3 large room temperature eggs	
2 teaspoons vanilla extract	*6* Let the cake cool completely on a wire rack and then slice the cake into two layers by slicing horizontally about 3 inches from the top.
2 tablespoons raw honey	
Shaved Paleo-friendly dark chocolate for garnish (optional)	*7* Spread the Chocolate Ganache over the bottom half of the cake and refrigerate for 30 minutes. Top with the other half of the cake and then spread the Chocolate Frosting over the top and sides of the cake.
	8 Sprinkle the top with shaved dark chocolate (if desired).

Chocolate Ganache

One 13.5-ounce can full-fat coconut milk

2 tablespoons raw honey

4 tablespoons raw cacao powder

½ teaspoon vanilla extract

1 In a medium saucepan, bring the coconut milk and honey to a light boil over medium heat; simmer uncovered on low for two hours, stirring occasionally, until the coconut milk reduces by half and becomes thicker and darker (similar to sweetened condensed milk).

2 Stir in the cacao powder and vanilla until all is combined and smooth.

3 Let it cool and refrigerate until it's thickened.

Chocolate Frosting

¾ cup Paleo-friendly dark chocolate chips

6 tablespoons full-fat coconut milk

1 Melt the chocolate chips in a bowl over simmering water (double boiler).

2 Mix the coconut milk with the melted chocolate until all is combined and smooth.

3 Let cool for 5 minutes before icing the cake.

Per serving: Calories 657 (From Fat 469); Fat 53g (Saturated 29g); Cholesterol 56mg; Sodium 550mg; Carbohydrate 44g (Dietary Fiber 9g); Protein 14g.

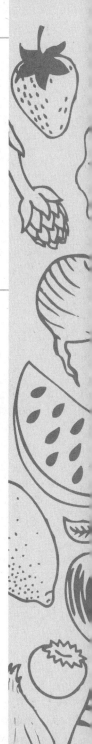

Coconut Chocolate Cake

Prep time: 30 min, plus chilling time • **Cook time:** 17 min • **Yield:** 10 servings

Ingredients	Directions
Coconut Layer (see the following recipe)	*1* Preheat the oven to 350 degrees. Lightly grease the bottom and sides of an 8-inch removable-bottom cake pan with coconut oil and cover the bottom of the pan with a cut piece of parchment paper.
Chocolate Glaze (see the following recipe)	
1½ cups blanched almond flour	*2* Mix the almond flour, cacao powder, coconut sugar, and salt.
½ cup raw cacao powder	
½ cup organic coconut palm sugar	*3* In a separate bowl whisk the eggs, coconut oil, coconut milk, and vanilla.
⅛ teaspoon salt	
2 room temperature eggs	*4* Using a rubber spatula, gently mix the dry ingredients and wet ingredients together. Mix just until ingredients are combined; don't overmix.
¼ cup coconut oil, melted	
⅓ cup full-fat coconut milk	*5* Spread the batter evenly in the pan and bake until a toothpick inserted into the center comes out clean, approximately 17 minutes. Cool on a wire rack.
2 teaspoons vanilla extract	
	6 Spread the Coconut Layer evenly over the cooled cake, followed by the Chocolate Glaze. Refrigerate for about 30 minutes or until the glaze is set. Keep refrigerated.

Coconut Layer

1½ cups unsweetened shredded coconut

1 tablespoon raw honey

⅓ cup blanched almond flour

¼ cup coconut oil, melted

¼ cup full-fat coconut milk

1 Mix all ingredients together until everything is well combined.

Chocolate Glaze

½ cup Paleo-friendly 70-percent dark chocolate

½ cup full-fat coconut milk

1 Slowly melt the dark chocolate in a bowl over simmering water (double boiler).

2 When the chocolate is melted, stir in the coconut milk and mix until the glaze is smooth.

Per serving: Calories 496 (From Fat 361); Fat 41g (Saturated 25g); Cholesterol 38mg; Sodium 69mg; Carbohydrate 28g (Dietary Fiber 6g); Protein 9g.

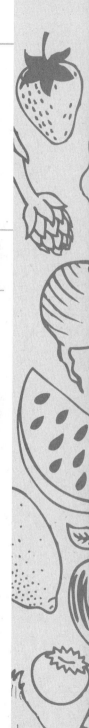

Banana Poppy Seed Cake with White Chocolate Vanilla Bean Frosting

Prep time: 30 min • **Cook time:** 30 min • **Yield:** 10 servings

Ingredients	Directions
White Chocolate Vanilla Bean Frosting (see the following recipe)	**1** Preheat the oven to 350 degrees. In a large bowl, mix the almond flour, flaxseed meal, tapioca flour, coconut sugar, baking soda, poppy seeds, and salt.
2 cups blanched almond flour	
¼ cup flaxseed meal	**2** Pulse the banana, coconut milk, coconut oil, eggs, and vanilla in a food processor until everything is combined.
¼ cup tapioca flour	
⅓ cup organic coconut palm sugar	**3** Using a rubber spatula, mix the dry ingredients and wet ingredients to form a batter. Don't overmix.
1 teaspoon baking soda	
1 tablespoon poppy seeds	**4** Line an 8-x-8-inch square baking pan with parchment paper, covering all four sides. Pour the batter evenly in the pan.
½ teaspoon salt	
1 cup mashed bananas	**5** Bake until a toothpick inserted into the center comes out clean, approximately 30 minutes.
½ cup full-fat coconut milk	
4 tablespoons coconut oil, melted	**6** Set the pan on a wire rack and allow the cake to cool. Spread the White Chocolate Vanilla Bean Frosting evenly over the cake.
2 room temperature eggs	
2 teaspoons vanilla extract	

White Chocolate Vanilla Bean Frosting

1 cup raw cashews

⅓ cup cacao butter, shaved into small pieces

1 tablespoon maple syrup

Seeds from 1 vanilla bean

1 teaspoon fresh lemon juice

Pinch of salt

2 to 4 tablespoons full-ft coconut milk

1 Process the cashews, cacao butter, maple syrup, vanilla bean seeds, lemon juice, and salt in a food processor until creamy and smooth.

2 Add the coconut milk 1 tablespoon at a time until the frosting reaches your desired consistency.

Tip: You can use your milk of choice or water as the liquid in the frosting recipe.

Per serving: Calories 426 (From Fat 298); Fat 33g (Saturated 13g); Cholesterol 37mg; Sodium 288mg; Carbohydrate 26g (Dietary Fiber 4g); Protein 9g.

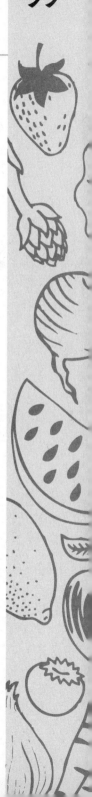

Carrot Cake with Chocolate Ganache

Prep time: 25 min • **Cook time:** 30–35 min • **Yield:** 10–12 servings

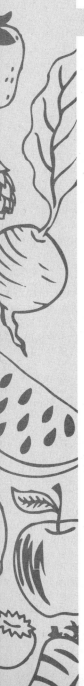

Ingredients	*Directions*
Easy Chocolate Ganache (see the following recipe)	*1* Preheat the oven to 350 degrees. In a large bowl, mix the almond flour, baking soda, coconut sugar, and chopped pecans.
3 cups blanched almond flour	
2 teaspoons baking soda	*2* In a separate bowl, whisk the eggs, coconut oil, vanilla, and carrots.
½ cup organic coconut palm sugar	
1 cup raw pecans, chopped	*3* Gently mix the wet ingredients and dry ingredients, using a rubber spatula. Don't overmix, or the almond flour will become oily.
3 room temperature eggs	
½ cup coconut oil, melted	*4* Lightly grease the bottom and sides of a round 8-inch removable-bottom cake pan with coconut oil and then cover the bottom of the pan with a piece of parchment paper. You don't need to fully grease the bottom. You can just put a few dots on the bottom to have the parchment stick or if you have pre-cut rounds, they lie flat perfectly and nothing else is needed.
2 teaspoons vanilla extract	
2 cups finely grated carrots (about 3 medium carrots)	
	5 Pour the batter evenly in the pan and bake until a toothpick inserted into the center comes out clean, approximately 30 to 35 minutes.
	6 Let the cake cool on a wire rack before removing it from the pan. Pour the Easy Chocolate Ganache over the cooled cake. Keep refrigerated.

Easy Chocolate Ganache

3 tablespoons coconut oil, melted

2 tablespoons raw cacao powder

1 tablespoon raw honey

3 tablespoons full-fat coconut milk

1 teaspoon vanilla extract

1 teaspoon arrowroot powder

1 Mix all the ingredients in a bowl over simmering water (double boiler) until combined and thickened.

Per serving: Calories 489 (From Fat 368); Fat 42g (Saturated 16g); Cholesterol 56mg; Sodium 310mg; Carbohydrate 26g (Dietary Fiber 6g); Protein 11g.

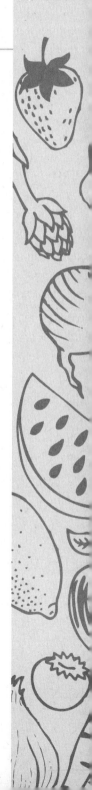

Orange Cake

Prep time: 15 min • **Cook time:** 35–40 min • **Yield:** 10–12 servings

Ingredients	Directions
6 eggs	*1* Preheat the oven to 350 degrees. Grease a round or square 8-inch pan with butter or coconut oil and line the bottom with parchment paper.
¼ cup coconut oil, melted	
¼ cup full-fat coconut milk	
2 tablespoons raw honey	*2* Whisk the eggs, coconut oil, coconut milk, honey, vanilla, and orange zest, reserving a bit of the zest for garnish (if desired).
1 teaspoon vanilla extract	
Zest of 1 orange	
½ cup coconut flour	*3* In a separate bowl, mix the coconut flour, baking soda, and sea salt.
½ teaspoon baking soda	
½ teaspoon salt	*4* Using a rubber spatula, mix the wet ingredients and dry ingredients.
Juice of ½ a medium orange (about ⅓ cup)	
Additional zest, for serving	*5* Pour the batter into the prepared pan and bake for 35 to 40 minutes or until a toothpick inserted into the center comes out clean. Cool on a wire rack.
	6 While the cake is still warm, poke holes all over the top with a fork and pour the orange juice evenly over the whole cake. Sprinkle the top with the reserved orange zest (if desired).

Per serving: Calories 141 (From Fat 90); Fat 10g (Saturated 8g); Cholesterol 112mg; Sodium 235mg; Carbohydrate 8g (Dietary Fiber 2g); Protein 5g.

Coconut Pie with Blueberries

Prep time: 25 min • **Cook time:** 5 min • **Yield:** 9 servings

Ingredients	Directions
Coconut Filling (see the following recipe)	*1* Chop the almonds and pecans separately in a food processor and place them in a large bowl.
½ cup raw almonds	
½ cup raw pecans	*2* Mix the date paste and chopped nuts with your hands until fully combined.
½ cup Medjool dates (about 6 large dates), pitted	*3* Line the bottom and sides of an 8-inch square (or round) pan with parchment paper and press the crust evenly across the bottom of the pan.
1 cup fresh blueberries	
	4 Pour the Coconut Filling over the crust. Refrigerate until the filling is firm and then cut the pie into squares and top it with fresh blueberries. Keep refrigerated.

Coconut Filling

1 can full-fat coconut milk	*1* Add the coconut milk and gelatin to a medium sauce pan and let it sit for 5 minutes.
1¼ teaspoon unflavored powdered gelatin	
2 tablespoons organic coconut palm sugar	*2* Heat the mixture over medium heat, stirring frequently until the gelatin is completely dissolved.
Pinch of salt	*3* Add the coconut sugar and salt and mix until the sugar dissolves. Mix in the shredded coconut and vanilla.
⅓ cup unsweetened shredded coconut	
½ teaspoon vanilla extract	

Tip: If the dates seem dry at all, I suggest a quick (5 minute) soak in hot water before making the paste; you want the paste to be as gooey as possible.

Per serving: Calories 221 (From Fat 145); Fat 16g (Saturated 8g); Cholesterol 0mg; Sodium 31mg; Carbohydrate 19g (Dietary Fiber 3g); Protein 3g.

Raspberry Chocolate Truffle Pie

Prep time: 30 min, plus overnight • **Cook time:** 5 min • **Yield:** 10 servings

Ingredients	*Directions*
Raspberry Filling (see the following recipe)	*1* Lightly grease the bottom and sides of a round 8-inch removable bottom cake pan with coconut oil and cover the bottom with a piece of parchment paper. As with others, the parchment just sits on the bottom fine.
½ **cup raw almonds**	
½ **cup raw pecans**	*2* Chop almonds and pecans in a food processor until coarse and place them in a bowl. Process the dates in the food processor until they form a creamy paste.
½ **cup Medjool dates (about 6 large dates), pitted**	
3 tablespoons raw cacao powder	*3* Add the date paste, cacao powder, coconut oil, and vanilla to the ground nuts and mix to combine all ingredients. Pat the crust mixture onto the bottom of the prepared pan.
½ **tablespoon coconut oil, melted**	
½ **teaspoon vanilla extract**	*4* Pour the Chocolate Raspberry Filling over the crust and freeze overnight. Remove the pie from the freezer, top with the raspberry sauce from the filling recipe, and serve. Store in the freezer.

Chocolate Raspberry Filling

1½ cup raspberries, fresh or frozen and thawed

One 13.5-ounce can full-fat coconut milk

3 tablespoons coconut oil, melted

1 cup Paleo-friendly chocolate chips

1 tablespoon vanilla extract

1 Pulse 1 cup of the raspberries in a food processor until smooth. Pour the puree into a strainer set over a bowl and gently press the raspberries to extract their juices.

2 Reserve ⅓ cup of the juice and mix the remaining juice with the remaining ½ cup of whole raspberries. Refrigerate until ready to serve.

3 Heat the coconut milk and coconut oil in a saucepan over medium heat until it starts to bubble. Remove the pan from the stove and mix in the reserved ⅓ cup raspberry juice, the chocolate chips, and the vanilla until the chocolate melts and everything is combined.

Per serving: Calories 368 (From Fat 245); Fat 27g (Saturated 16g); Cholesterol 0mg; Sodium 15mg; Carbohydrate 31g (Dietary Fiber 4g); Protein 5g.

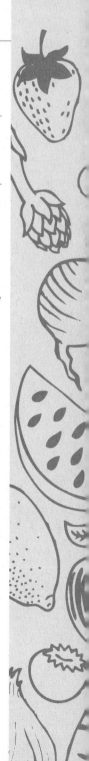

Mini No-bake Blueberry Cheesecakes

Prep time: 25 min, plus overnight • **Cook time:** 30 min • **Yield:** 10 servings

Ingredients	Directions
⅓ cup pecans	*1* Chop the almonds in a food processor and set aside in a bowl. Process the pecans and add them to the almonds.
⅓ cup almonds	
5 large Medjool dates, pitted	*2* Process the dates in the food processor until they're creamy and then mix the date paste into the almonds and pecans.
2 cups raw cashews	
2 tablespoons coconut oil, melted	*3* Press 1 tablespoon of the mixture into each individual cavity of a mini removable-bottom cheesecake pan and press down to flatten crust.
½ cup plus 2 tablespoons plain Greek yogurt	
¼ cup lemon juice	*4* Process the cashews and coconut oil in the food processor until creamy. In a large bowl, mix this cashew butter with the remaining ingredients; pour the mixture into the crusts and freeze overnight.
2 tablespoons raw honey	
Pinch of salt	
	5 Unmold each cheesecake and drizzle with the Blueberry Sauce and serve. Store any leftover cheesecakes in the freezer.

Blueberry Sauce

2 cups blueberries (fresh or frozen and thawed)	**1** Bring all the ingredients to a boil in a saucepan over medium heat.
⅔ cup water	
1 teaspoon lemon juice	**2** Mash the blueberries and simmer for about 30 minutes at medium-low heat.
	3 Store blueberry sauce in the fridge to preserve.

Tip: You can use 1 cup of cashew butter in place of the raw cashews.

Vary It! Replace the Greek yogurt with the coconut cream from a can of chilled coconut milk. (Refrigerate a can of coconut milk for at least 12 hours; the cream is what you scoop off the top, discarding the water.)

Vary It! If you don't have mini cheesecake pans, you can make this recipe in a muffin tin. Line your tin with paper muffin cups for easy removal.

Per serving: Calories 270 (From Fat 157); Fat 18g (Saturated 5g); Cholesterol 1mg; Sodium 27mg; Carbohydrate 24g (Dietary Fiber 3g); Protein 7g.

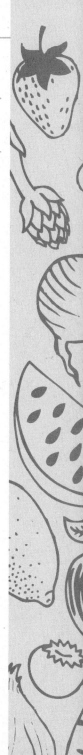

Coconut Cream Pie

Prep time: 35 min • **Cook time:** 25 min • **Yield:** 8 servings

Ingredients	Directions
Coconut Cream Layer (see the following recipe)	*1* Preheat the oven to 350 degrees. Line the bottom and sides of a 7-x-5-inch baking pan with parchment paper.
¼ **cup pecans, chopped**	
½ **cup blanched almond flour**	*2* In a large bowl, mix the pecans, almond flour, honey, and coconut oil.
½ **tablespoon raw honey**	
3 tablespoons coconut oil, melted	*3* Press mixture onto the bottom of the prepared baking pan and bake for about 10 minutes or until the top and edges start to brown. Cool on a wire rack.
6 tablespoons Paleo-friendly chocolate chips	*4* Melt the chocolate chips slowly in a bowl over simmering water (double boiler). When the chocolate is melted, mix in the coconut milk. Spread the mixture evenly over the cooled crust and refrigerate.
1 tablespoon plus 1 teaspoon full-fat coconut milk	
One 13.5-ounce can full-fat coconut milk, chilled overnight	*5* Pour the Coconut Cream Layer over the chocolate and refrigerate until the coconut layer is firm.
Toasted unsweetened shredded coconut for garnish	*6* Scoop the cream from the chilled can of coconut milk into a large bowl, discarding the water. Whip the cream with a handheld or stand mixer until fluffy and then spread it over the Coconut Cream Layer.
	7 Sprinkle the top with the toasted coconut.

Coconut Cream Layer

One 13.5-ounce can full-fat coconut milk

1 large egg

3 tablespoons arrowroot powder

3 tablespoons raw honey

⅛ teaspoon salt

½ teaspoon vanilla extract

½ cup unsweetened shredded coconut

1 Combine the coconut milk, egg, arrowroot powder, honey, and salt in a saucepan. Heat the mixture slowly over medium heat, stirring constantly until it thickens.

2 Remove the mixture from the stove and stir in the vanilla and shredded coconut.

Per serving: Calories 571 (From Fat 434); Fat 49g (Saturated 34g); Cholesterol 36mg; Sodium 99mg; Carbohydrate 32g (Dietary Fiber 3g); Protein 7g.

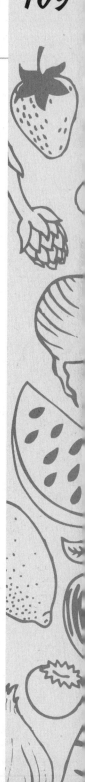

Coconut Cream Pie with Strawberries

Prep time: 20 min, plus overnight • **Cook time:** 5 min • **Yield:** 8 servings

Ingredients	*Directions*
Coconut Cream (see the following recipe)	**1** Process the dates in a food processor until a creamy paste forms. Mix the date paste with the remaining ingredients and press the mixture evenly on the bottom and sides of two 4.75-inch removable-bottom tart pans.
½ cup Medjool dates (about 6 large dates), pitted	
⅓ cup pecans, chopped	**2** Pour the Coconut Cream evenly over each crust and refrigerate overnight or until the coconut cream layer is set.
½ cup blanched almond flour	
4 tablespoons raw cacao powder	
½ teaspoon vanilla extract	**3** Garnish with the fresh strawberries and drizzle with the melted dark chocolate before serving.
1 cup fresh strawberries, sliced	
¼ cup melted Paleo-friendly dark chocolate for garnish	

Coconut Cream

One 13.5-ounce can full-fat coconut milk

1 large egg

3 tablespoons arrowroot powder

3 tablespoons raw honey

⅛ teaspoon salt

½ teaspoon vanilla extract

½ cup unsweetened shredded coconut

1 In a saucepan, whisk the coconut milk, egg, arrowroot powder, honey, and salt.

2 Heat the mixture slowly over medium heat, stirring constantly until it thickens.

3 Let the mixture cool for 5 minutes and then mix in the vanilla and shredded coconut.

Tip: Mix in some of the coconut "water" from the can that you took the cream out of and add that into the melted chocolate to thin it bit and make it more drizzly.

Per serving: Calories 310 (From Fat 183); Fat 20g (Saturated 12g); Cholesterol 0mg; Sodium 67mg; Carbohydrate 31g (Dietary Fiber 5g); Protein 5g.

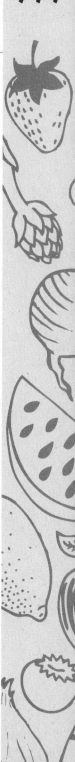

No-bake Macadamia Nut Pie

Prep time: 20 min, plus freezing time • **Yield:** 10 servings

Ingredients	Directions
Macadamia Filling (see the following recipe)	*1* Line the bottom of a round 8-inch removable-bottom pan with parchment paper.
½ cup pecans, chopped	
½ cup unsweetened shredded coconut	*2* In a bowl, combine the pecans, shredded coconut, almond flour, coconut oil, honey, and cacao powder. Work the mixture with your hands until all ingredients are combined and a dough forms.
1 cup blanched almond flour	
5 tablespoons coconut oil, melted	
1 tablespoon raw honey	*3* Pat the crust mixture onto the bottom of the prepared pan. Pour the Macadamia Filling over the crust.
2 tablespoons raw cacao powder	
½ cup macadamia nuts, chopped	*4* Sprinkle the top with the chopped macadamia nuts and freeze for about 4 hours before serving. Keep frozen.

Macadamia Filling

1 cup macadamia nut butter

6 large Medjool dates, pitted

1 cup plain full-fat Greek yogurt

4 tablespoons coconut oil, melted

1 tablespoon vanilla extract

1 teaspoon fresh orange juice

Pinch of salt

1 Process the dates in a blender or food processor until smooth.

2 Add the remaining ingredients and process until smooth.

Tip: You can save money by making your own macadamia nut butter. Process 2¼ cups of macadamia nuts in your food processor for a few minutes, scraping the sides as needed, until the nuts are creamy and smooth.

Vary It! Replace the Greek yogurt with full fat yogurt or the coconut cream from a can of chilled coconut milk. (Refrigerate a can of coconut milk overnight; the cream is what you scoop off the top, discarding the water.) You can also use lemon juice in place of the orange juice.

Per serving: Calories 535 (From Fat 441); Fat 50g (Saturated 18g); Cholesterol 0mg; Sodium 1mg; Carbohydrate 22g (Dietary Fiber 6g); Protein 9g.

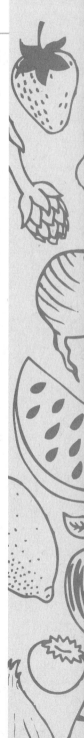

Chocolate Hazelnut Pie

Prep time: 20 min, plus freezing time • **Yield:** 10 servings

Ingredients	Directions
Hazelnut Filling (see the following recipe)	**1** Line the bottom of a round 8-inch removable-bottom pan with parchment paper.
6 large Medjool dates, pitted	**2** Process the dates in a blender or food processor until creamy and smooth. Add the remaining ingredients and pulse to combine.
¾ cup pecans, chopped	
¾ cup unsweetened shredded coconut	
2 tablespoons pastured butter	**3** Spread the mixture evenly onto the bottom of the prepared pan. Pour the Hazelnut Filling over the crust and freeze for about 4 hours. Keep frozen.
1 teaspoon vanilla extract	

Hazelnut Filling

6 large Medjool dates, pitted	**1** In a blender or food processor, process the dates until creamy and smooth.
1 cup hazelnut butter	
4 tablespoons coconut oil, melted	**2** Add the remaining ingredients and process until smooth.
1 cup plain full-fat Greek yogurt	
4 tablespoons raw cacao powder	
1 tablespoon vanilla extract	
Pinch of salt	

Tip: You can save money by making your own hazelnut butter. Process 2-¼ cups of blanched hazelnuts in your food processor for a few minutes, scraping the sides as needed, until the nuts are creamy and smooth.

Vary It! Replace the Greek yogurt with the coconut cream from a can of chilled coconut milk. (Refrigerate a can of coconut milk overnight; the cream is what you scoop off the top, discarding the water.)

Per serving: Calories 413 (From Fat 282); Fat 32g (Saturated 12g); Cholesterol 7mg; Sodium 33mg; Carbohydrate 27g (Dietary Fiber 7g); Protein 9g.

Mixed-Berry Pie with Sweet Coconut Whipped Cream

Prep time: 35 min, plus overnight • **Cook time:** 12 min • **Yield:** 10–12 servings

Ingredients	Directions
Sweet Coconut Whipped Cream (see the following recipe)	*1* Preheat the oven to 350 degrees. Grease the bottom and sides of a round 8-inch removable-bottom tart pan and line the bottom with parchment paper
½ cup unsweetened shredded coconut 1 cup blanched almond flour ½ cup pecans, finely chopped	*2* In a large bowl, mix the shredded coconut, almond flour, pecans, coconut oil, and 1 tablespoon of the honey.
6 tablespoons coconut oil, melted 1 tablespoon raw honey	*3* Pat the dough onto the bottom and sides of the prepared pan. Bake for 12 minutes or until crust starts to brown. Cool on a wire rack.
½ cup Sugar-Free Strawberry Jam 2 cups strawberries, raspberries, blueberries, and/or cherries, fresh or frozen and thawed 1 cup fresh raspberries	*4* Mix the jam with the berries. Pour the mixture over the crust and top it with the fresh raspberries. Refrigerate for about 5 hours and top with the Sweet Coconut Whipped Cream before serving.

Sweet Coconut Whipped Cream

1 can 13.5 ounces full-fat coconut milk 1 tablespoon raw honey	*1* Chill the can of coconut milk overnight. Scoop the solid coconut cream from the top of the can into a bowl, discarding the water.
½ teaspoon vanilla extract	*2* Add the honey and vanilla and whip the mixture with an electric mixer until fluffy.

Tip: You can find the recipe for Sugar-Free Strawberry Jam in Chapter 11.

Per serving: *Calories 275 (From Fat 224); Fat 25g (Saturated 14g); Cholesterol 0mg; Sodium 9mg; Carbohydrate 13g (Dietary Fiber 3g); Protein 4g.*

Mini Raspberry Chocolate Tarts

Prep time: 30 min, plus chilling time • **Cook time:** 15 minutes plus 2 hours • **Yield:** 9 servings

Ingredients	*Directions*
Chocolate Filling (see the following recipe)	*1* Preheat the oven to 350. Using a rubber spatula, mix the pecans, almond flour, honey, and coconut oil.
½ cup pecans, finely chopped	
1 cup blanched almond flour	*2* Press the mixture onto the bottom and sides of individual cavity of a 9-cup silicon or nonstick muffin pan. (If you're using a nonstick muffin pan, line each cavity with paper liners.)
1 tablespoon raw honey	
6 tablespoons coconut oil, melted	
1 cup fresh raspberries	*3* Bake for about 12 minutes or until the crust starts to turn brown.
	4 Fill the baked crusts with the Chocolate Filling and top them with the fresh raspberries. Chill the tarts in the fridge for about 4 hours before serving.

Chocolate Filling

One 13.5-ounce can full-fat coconut milk	*1* Bring the coconut milk and honey to a light boil over medium heat.
3 tablespoons raw honey	
4 tablespoons raw cacao powder	*2* Lower the heat to low and cook for about 2 hours, stirring occasionally, until it's thick enough that it doesn't run off the spoon easily and has a consistency similar to sweetened condensed milk.
½ teaspoon vanilla extract	
	3 Stir in the cacao powder and vanilla.
	4 Raise the heat to medium and cook for another 7 minutes, stirring frequently and scraping the sides of the pan. Remove the pan from the heat, and let the mixture cool completely.

Per serving: Calories 323 (From Fat 260); Fat 29g (Saturated 17g); Cholesterol 0mg; Sodium 12mg; Carbohydrate 16g (Dietary Fiber 3g); Protein 5g.

Chocolate Haupia Pie

Prep time: 25 min, plus overnight • **Cook time:** 5 min • **Yield:** 10 servings

Ingredients	*Directions*
Haupia (see the following recipe)	*1* Line the bottom and sides of a square 8-x-8-inch pan with parchment paper.
⅔ cup raw almonds	
⅔ cup raw pecans	*2* Grind the almonds and pecans separately in a food processor until they're coarse ground.
1 cup Medjool dates (about 10 large dates), pitted	*3* Process the dates in the food processor until they're creamy. Mix the nuts and date paste by hand until well combined; press the mixture evenly onto the bottom of the prepared pan.
6 tablespoons raw cacao powder	
¼ cup chopped 70-percent Paleo-friendly dark chocolate, or chocolate chips	*4* Pour the Haupia over the crust and refrigerate overnight or until the filling is firm. Cut into squares. Melt the dark chocolate in a bowl over simmering water (double boiler) then drizzle chocolate over each square before serving.

Haupia

½ cup arrowroot powder	*1* Mix the arrowroot powder and water in a saucepan until the arrowroot is dissolved. Whisk in the coconut milk and honey.
¾ cup water	
1 can full-fat coconut milk	
2 tablespoons raw honey	*2* Cook the mixture over medium-low heat, stirring constantly, until it thickens, about 10 minutes.
½ teaspoon vanilla extract	
	3 Remove the mixture from the heat and stir in the vanilla.

Note: Haupia is a tradition Hawaiian dessert often eaten on its own or as a topping for chocolate mousse pies or wedding cakes. Haupia is traditionally made from coconut milk, sugar, coconut extract and a starch to thicken it. The consistency is similar to a gelatin or thick pudding. Some recipes also add additional fresh or dried shredded coconut to enhance that incredible coconut flavor.

Per serving: Calories 327 (From Fat 194); Fat 22g (Saturated 11g); Cholesterol 0mg; Sodium 12mg; Carbohydrate 36g (Dietary Fiber 5g); Protein 5g.

Chocolate Hazelnut Tart with Strawberries

Prep time: 25 min • **Yield:** 8 servings

Ingredients	Directions
Homemade Chocolate Hazelnut Spread (see the following recipe)	*1* Process the dates in a food processor until they form a creamy paste.
½ cup Medjool dates (about 6 large dates), pitted	*2* In a large bowl, mix the date paste, almond flour, pecans, and vanilla by hand.
½ cup blanched almond flour	
⅓ cup pecans, chopped	*3* Spread the mixture onto the bottom of two 4.75-inch removable-bottom tart pans.
½ teaspoon vanilla extract	
1½ cups fresh strawberries, sliced	*4* Pour the Homemade Chocolate Hazelnut Spread over the crust and top it with the fresh strawberries.

Homemade Chocolate Hazelnut Spread

3 tablespoons Paleo-friendly chocolate chips

1 cup hazelnut butter

2 tablespoons full-fat coconut milk

2 tablespoons raw cacao powder

3 tablespoons coconut oil, melted

1 tablespoon organic coconut palm sugar

½ teaspoon vanilla extract

Pinch of salt

1 Melt the chocolate chips in a bowl over simmering water (double boiler). Remove from heat and stir in the remaining ingredients.

Tip: You can substitute pastured heavy cream for the coconut milk in the hazelnut spread.

Tip: You can save money by making your own hazelnut butter. Process 2¼ cups of blanched hazelnuts in your food processor for a few minutes, scraping the sides as needed, until the nuts are creamy and smooth.

Per serving: *Calories 403 (From Fat 278); Fat 31g (Saturated 8g); Cholesterol 0mg; Sodium 26mg; Carbohydrate 28g (Dietary Fiber 8g); Protein 8g.*

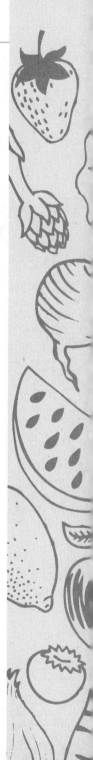

Chapter 7

Decadent Chocolates and Truffles

In This Chapter

▶ Discovering the healthy aspects of chocolate

▶ Creating rich, yummy treats

I love, love, love chocolate! I'm guessing you do, too (or know someone who does), so this chapter is full of delicious chocolate treat recipes for the health-conscious chocolate lover.

The striking difference you notice with these recipes is that everything is made with healthy fats and protein, and sweetened only slightly with natural sweeteners such as raw honey and coconut palm sugar. None of the recipes contains refined white flours or sugars, artificial sweeteners, soy, or chemicals. Best of all, the recipes are easy to make, taste amazing, and don't require you to own a candy factory. Paleo recipes *never* sacrifice taste!

Did you know that the cacao plant produces one of nature's superfoods? Raw cacao beans are high in antioxidants; minerals such as calcium, magnesium, potassium, and manganese; and healthy fats.

Cacao's health benefits are one of the reasons Paleo advocates love a chocolate treat. However, not all chocolate is the same. Adding loads of sugar and milk degrades the quality of the chocolate and blocks the absorption of the nutrients you're hoping to take in. High-cacao dark chocolate, with a minimum of 70 percent cacao (and no soy), is what you should look for. It's dark, rich, bitter, and delicious. "Bitter" and "delicious" may sound like a contradiction in terms, but after you've purged your taste buds of chemically hyper-flavored, over-salted, and super-sweetened foods, you discover a whole host of flavors hidden beneath those top notes. One of my favorite brands of dark chocolate is by Equal Exchange.

Raw cacao powder isn't the same as natural cocoa or Dutch-processed cocoa powder. Raw cacao powder contains the highest amounts of beneficial anti-oxidants and minerals by far, and it tastes much better and less bitter. My favorite raw cacao powder is made by Essential Living Foods.

The recipes in this chapter often call for Paleo-friendly chocolate chips. I prefer chocolate chips from the Enjoy Life brand; they're Paleo-approved chocolate chips that are dairy-, nut-, and soy-free. But whenever a recipe calls for chocolate chips, you can substitute any Paleo-friendly chocolate bar chopped into small pieces, or you can make your own chocolate chips from the 84-Percent Dark Chocolate Sweetened with Honey recipe in this chapter.

84-Percent Dark Chocolate Sweetened with Honey

Prep time: 30 min, plus cooling • **Cook time:** 5 min • **Yield:** 9 servings

Ingredients	Directions
2½ tablespoons cacao butter	*1* Melt the cacao butter in a bowl over simmering water (double boiler) until it reaches 122 degrees.
3½ tablespoons raw cacao powder	*2* Add the cacao powder, honey, and vanilla. Mix until the ingredients are combined and the mixture reaches 122 degrees.
1 tablespoon raw honey	
¼ teaspoon vanilla extract	*3* Begin tempering the chocolate by pouring the mixture on a chilled marble slab or glass cutting board.
	4 With a flexible plastic scraper or palette knife, spread the chocolate thinly, scoop it up, and spread it again. Repeat the sequence, keeping the chocolate constantly on the move for about 5 to10 minutes or until the chocolate sets quickly when dropping a little of the onto the side of the slab/board. The chocolate setting quickly is a sign it's tempered and ready to pour into molds.
	5 Let the tempered chocolate cool at room temperature for a few hours.

Per one-ounce serving: Calories 126 (From Fat 94); Fat 11g (Saturated 7g); Cholesterol 0mg; Sodium 3mg; Carbohydrate 7g (Dietary Fiber 1g); Protein 1g.

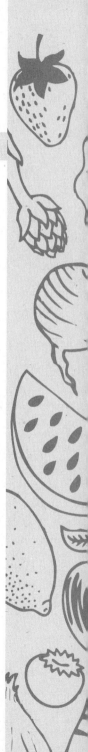

Raspberry-Filled Homemade Chocolates

Prep time: 10 min, plus freezing time • **Cook time:** 5 min • **Yield:** 15 servings

Ingredients	*Directions*
2 tablespoons almond butter	**1** Whisk the almond butter, coconut oil, cacao powder, vanilla, and salt in a bowl over simmering water (double boiler) until melted and combined.
3 tablespoons coconut oil, melted	
3 tablespoons raw cacao powder	**2** Halfway fill 15 cavities of a silicone candy mold with the melted chocolate.
½ teaspoon vanilla extract	
Pinch of salt	**3** Add 1 raspberry to each cavity and cover with more chocolate.
1 tablespoon raw honey	
15 frozen or fresh raspberries	**4** Freeze until the chocolate is set, about 20 minutes. Store in the freezer or fridge.

Per serving: *Calories 49 (From Fat 38); Fat 4g (Saturated 3g); Cholesterol 0mg; Sodium 15mg; Carbohydrate 2g (Dietary Fiber 1g); Protein 1g.*

Chocolate Pecan Crunch Truffles

Prep time: 15 min • **Cook time:** 5 min • **Yield:** 18 servings

Ingredients	Directions
3 tablespoons cacao paste, chopped	**1** Melt the cacao paste in a bowl over simmering water (double boiler).
⅔ cup raw pecans, finely chopped	**2** Whisk the melted cacao paste with the pecans, coconut butter, honey, vanilla, and salt.
4 tablespoons coconut butter, melted	
1 tablespoon raw honey	**3** Using your hands, shape the mixture into 1-inch balls (the mixture may be crumbly). Place each of these truffles on a cookie sheet with parchment paper and freeze for 20 minutes.
½ teaspoon vanilla extract	
Pinch of salt	
3 tablespoons cacao butter	**4** Melt the cacao butter and chocolate chips in another bowl over simmering water (double boiler).
3 tablespoons Paleo-friendly chocolate chips	
	5 Using a fork, dip each truffle time in the melted chocolate and place it back on the parchment paper. Refrigerate until chocolate sets.

Tip: You can use 100-percent unsweetened dark chocolate in place of the cacao paste in Step 1 and coconut oil in place of the cacao butter in Step 4.

Tip: Melt the coconut butter before using it, and be sure to stir the content in the jar before measuring. You can melt the coconut butter by placing the jar in a saucepan with water and heating it over medium-low heat.

Per serving: Calories 99 (From Fat 81); Fat 9g (Saturated 5g); Cholesterol 0mg; Sodium 10mg; Carbohydrate 4g (Dietary Fiber 1g); Protein 1g.

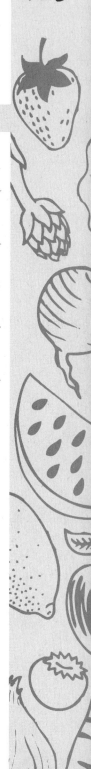

Paleo Chocolate Caramel Wafer Bars

Prep time: 30 min, plus chilling time • **Cook time:** 10–15 min • **Yield:** 14 servings

Ingredients	Directions
Caramel Sauce (see the following recipe)	**1** Preheat the oven to 350 degrees. In a large bowl, mix the almond flour, arrowroot powder, and salt.
½ cup plus 6 tablespoons blanched almond flour	**2** In a separate bowl, whisk the coconut oil, vanilla, and honey.
¼ cup arrowroot powder	
Pinch of salt	**3** Using a rubber spatula, gently mix the wet ingredients and dry ingredients together. Don't overmix.
4 tablespoons coconut oil, melted	**4** Line a cookie sheet with parchment paper, and shape the dough into a 6-x-7-inch square of about ¼-inch thickness. Bake for 10 to 15 minutes or until the edges and top start to brown.
1½ teaspoons vanilla extract	
1 tablespoon raw honey	
½ cup Paleo-friendly dark chocolate chips	**5** Remove the cookie from the oven and immediately cut it into approximately fourteen 1-x-3-inch pieces with a knife or pastry chopper (using a serrated knife minimizes crumbling). Don't separate the pieces. Set the cookie sheet on a wire rack to cool and then separate each piece.
1 tablespoon cacao butter	
	6 Spread the Caramel Layer evenly across the top of each cooled cookie. Refrigerate until the caramel hardens.
	7 Melt the chocolate chips and cacao butter slowly in a bowl over simmering water (double boiler). Dip each cookie in the melted chocolate; lay the cookies on parchment paper and refrigerate until set. Store in an airtight container in the fridge.

Caramel Layer

2 tablespoons water

¼ cup organic coconut palm sugar

½ cup full-fat coconut milk

1 teaspoon vanilla extract

Pinch of salt

1 Bring the water and coconut sugar to a boil, stirring the mixture constantly over medium heat.

2 Add the remaining ingredients and cook for about 10 minutes over medium heat, stirring constantly so that it doesn't burn. The mixture will start to thicken and turn darker.

Tip: If you're a fan of Mars-brand Twix bars, this recipe is a great Paleo substitute.

Per serving: Calories 173 (From Fat 118); Fat 13g (Saturated 8g); Cholesterol 0mg; Sodium 27mg; Carbohydrate 15g (Dietary Fiber 2g); Protein 2g.

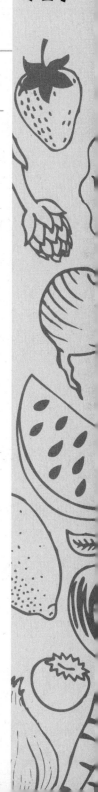

Hot Chocolate on a Stick

Prep time: 10 min, plus chilling time • **Cook time:** 5 min • **Yield:** 3 servings

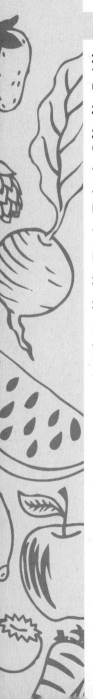

Ingredients	*Directions*
3½ tablespoons Paleo-friendly 100-percent dark unsweetened chocolate	**1** Melt the chocolate and cacao butter in a bowl over simmering water (double boiler). Whisk in the coconut sugar, honey, ground vanilla, coffee, and salt until well combined.
2½ tablespoons cacao butter	
2 tablespoons organic coconut palm sugar	
1 tablespoon raw honey	**2** Pour the chocolate into silicone ice cube trays and refrigerate until it's set around the edges but still soft in the center (about 10 minutes). Insert a wooden stick in the center of each cube and refrigerate until the chocolate has hardened completely before removing the mold.
¼ teaspoon ground vanilla bean	
1 teaspoon instant coffee	
Pinch of salt	**3** Keep the chocolate sticks refrigerated. To make a hot chocolate drink, heat the almond milk and then swirl the chocolate around to dissolve.
3 wooden popsicle sticks	
3 cups almond milk	

Vary It! Substitute your Paleo-friendly milk of choice — raw milk, coconut milk, or whatever your preference — in Step 3.

Per serving: Calories 247 (From Fat 185); Fat 21g (Saturated 14g); Cholesterol 0mg; Sodium 53mg; Carbohydrate 20g (Dietary Fiber 3g); Protein 2g. (Analysis does not include milk.)

Chocolate-Covered "Peanut Butter" Pops

Prep time: 25 min, plus freezing time • **Yield:** 12 servings

Ingredients	*Directions*
12 tablespoons blanched almond flour	*1* Using a rubber spatula, mix the almond flour, flaxseed meal, salt, butter, coconut milk, vanilla, and sunflower seed butter until combined. Don't overmix.
2 tablespoon flaxseed meal	
⅛ teaspoons of salt	
2½ tablespoons pastured butter, softened	*2* Line an 8½-x-4½-inch medium loaf pan with parchment paper and pack the mixture across the bottom of the pan.
1 tablespoon full-fat coconut milk	
2 teaspoon vanilla extract	*3* Place pan in the freezer until the mixture is set; then cut it into squares of about 1½ inches.
6 tablespoons sunflower seed butter	*4* Allow the squares to warm up for 5 minutes and then insert a stick halfway into each square. Keep the pops frozen until you're ready to dip them in chocolate.
12 lollypop sticks	
⅔ cup Paleo-friendly chocolate chips	*5* Melt the chocolate chips and coconut oil in a bowl over simmering water (double boiler) and then dip each square in the melted chocolate. Store in an airtight container in the fridge.
4 teaspoons coconut oil, melted	

Tip: Stir the content in the jar of sunflower seed butter before measuring.

Per serving: Calories 204 (From Fat 150); Fat 17g (Saturated 6g); Cholesterol 6mg; Sodium 53mg; Carbohydrate 12g (Dietary Fiber 2g); Protein 4g.

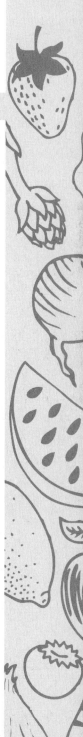

Coconut Dream Cups

Prep time: 20 min, plus chilling time • **Yield:** 6 servings

Ingredients	Directions
¼ cup coconut butter, melted	**1** Place two teaspoons of the coconut butter into each of six silicone cup molds and refrigerate for about 10 minutes.
3½ tablespoons Paleo-friendly 100-percent dark unsweetened chocolate	
1 tablespoon raw cacao powder	**2** Melt the chocolate in a bowl over simmering water (double boiler) and stir in the cacao powder, coconut milk, vanilla, honey, and salt.
2½ tablespoons full-fat coconut milk	
¼ teaspoon vanilla extract	**3** Add one teaspoon of the chocolate to the center of each cup and refrigerate until the chocolate is set.
2½ tablespoons raw honey	**4** Add one more teaspoon of the chocolate to the center and refrigerate again until set.
Pinch of salt	
Unsweetened coconut flakes for garnish	**5** Top each cup with two teaspoons of the remaining coconut butter and refrigerate until set. Garnish with the coconut flakes and serve. Store in an airtight container in the fridge.

Tip: If your coconut butter isn't soft, melt it by putting the jar in a saucepan, covering it with water, and heating it slowly until it melts completely. Stir the content in the jar before using. You can also make your own coconut butter: Process 1 cup of unsweetened dry shredded coconut in your food processor for a few minutes, scraping the sides as needed, until it's creamy and smooth.

Tip: You can skip Step 4 and just add 2 teaspoons of chocolate in Step 3 all at once; just know that if you take this route, the chocolate will spread to the sides and you'll see the line of chocolate on the sides of the cups.

Per serving: Calories 148 (From Fat 107); Fat 12g (Saturated 10g); Cholesterol 0mg; Sodium 29mg; Carbohydrate 12g (Dietary Fiber 3g); Protein 2g.

Cookie Dough Bites

Prep time: 10 min, plus freezing time • **Yield:** 12 servings

Ingredients	Directions
3 tablespoons coconut oil, melted	*1* Whisk together the coconut oil, coconut milk, vanilla, and honey.
1½ tablespoons full-fat coconut milk	*2* Using a rubber spatula, gently mix in the almond flour until the ingredients are combined. Be careful not to overmix, or the batter will become oily.
¾ teaspoon vanilla extract	
2 teaspoons raw honey	
¾ cup blanched almond flour	*3* Fold in 3 tablespoons of the chocolate chips and freeze the dough for about 20 minutes.
3 tablespoons Paleo-friendly chocolate chips, plus more for garnish (about 3 to 4 tablespoons)	*4* Roll chilled dough into 12 balls (2 teaspoons per ball) and place on a cookie sheet lined with parchment paper.
	5 Melt the remaining chocolate chips in a bowl over simmering water (double boiler).
	6 Drizzle the melted chocolate over each cookie dough bite. Store any leftover bites in the refrigerator.

Per serving: Calories 103 (From Fat 79); Fat 9g (Saturated 5g); Cholesterol 0mg; Sodium 3mg; Carbohydrate 6g (Dietary Fiber 1g); Protein 2g.

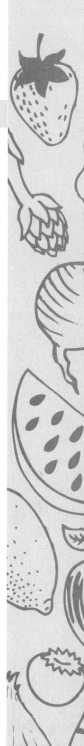

Homemade Coconut Almond Candy Bars

Prep time: 20 min, plus freezing time • **Yield:** 13 servings

Ingredients	Directions
1½ cups unsweetened shredded coconut	*1* In a large bowl, mix the shredded coconut, coconut oil, coconut butter, vanilla, honey, and salt.
¼ cup coconut oil, melted	
5 tablespoons coconut butter	*2* Line an 8½-x-4½-inch medium loaf pan with parchment paper and press the mixture onto the bottom of the pan.
1 teaspoon vanilla extract	
2 tablespoons raw honey	*3* Freeze the dough for about 30 minutes and then cut it into small (2-inch-x-1½-inch) rectangles. Return to the freezer.
Pinch of salt	
26 raw almonds	
½ cup cacao butter	*4* Melt the cacao butter and chocolate chips in a bowl over simmering water (double boiler) and then let the chocolate cool for 5 minutes.
½ cup Paleo-friendly chocolate chips	
	5 Remove the bars from the freezer and line a cookie sheet with parchment paper. Place two almonds on top of each coconut bar and dip each bar into the melted chocolate, using a fork.
	6 Refrigerate until the chocolate hardens. Store in an airtight container in the fridge.

Tip: For a thicker shell of chocolate, dip each bar in melted chocolate twice and refrigerate until chocolate hardens. You can also substitute melted coconut oil for the cacao butter in Step 4.

Tip: This recipe is a great Paleo-approved option for folks who enjoy Hershey's Almond Joy candy bars.

Per serving: Calories 296 (From Fat 243); Fat 27g (Saturated 20g); Cholesterol 0mg; Sodium 17mg; Carbohydrate 13g (Dietary Fiber 3g); Protein 2g.

Peppermint Chocolate Sticks

Prep time: 10 min • **Yield:** 10 servings

Ingredients	*Directions*
6 tablespoons coconut oil, melted	*1* In a large bowl, mix the coconut oil, cacao powder, almond butter, honey, vanilla, peppermint extract, and salt.
4 tablespoons raw cacao powder	
4 tablespoons almond butter	*2* Heat the mixture slowly on low heat over simmering water (double boiler) for 5 to 10 minutes until all ingredients are combined.
2 tablespoons raw honey	
1 teaspoon vanilla extract	
½ teaspoon peppermint extract	*3* Add the pecans and shredded coconut to the melted chocolate and stir.
Pinch of salt	
½ cup pecans, coarsely chopped	*4* Pour the chocolate into a 7-x-5-inch dish lined with parchment paper, making sure the paper covers all four sides of the pan.
½ cup unsweetened shredded coconut	
	5 Freeze until the chocolate is set, and then cut into sticks. Store in airtight container in freezer.

Per serving: Calories 204 (From Fat 168); Fat 19g (Saturated 11g); Cholesterol 0mg; Sodium 31mg; Carbohydrate 8g (Dietary Fiber 2g); Protein 3g.

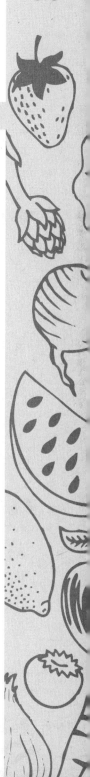

Strawberry-Banana Chocolate Cups

Prep time: 25 min, plus freezing time • **Yield:** 12 servings

Ingredients	Directions
⅔ cup chopped fresh strawberries	*1* Process the strawberries, banana, date, almond butter, and lemon juice in a food processor or high speed blender until creamy and smooth.
⅓ cup chopped banana	
1 large Medjool date, pitted	*2* Melt the chocolate slowly in a bowl over simmering water (double boiler).
1½ teaspoons almond butter	
¼ teaspoon fresh lemon juice	*3* Fill the bottom of mini silicon muffin cups with 1 teaspoon of the melted chocolate and freeze for 5 minutes.
1 cup Paleo-friendly dark chocolate	
	4 When the chocolate has hardened, top the center of each muffin cup with about ½ teaspoon of the strawberry-banana mixture and then freeze for another 5 minutes.
	5 Fill the cups ¾ of the way full with the remaining melted chocolate. Freeze until the chocolate is set. Store in an airtight container in the fridge for up to 1 week.

Vary It! You can replace the chocolate chips with 84-Percent Dark Chocolate Sweetened with Honey (see the recipe earlier in this chapter, and double it to get the 1 cup of chocolate required for this recipe).

Per serving: Calories 120 (From Fat 70); Fat 8g (Saturated 4g); Cholesterol 0mg; Sodium 6mg; Carbohydrate 12g (Dietary Fiber 2g); Protein 2g.

Homemade Hazelnut Chocolates

Prep time: 25 min, plus chilling time • **Cook time:** 5 min • **Yield:** 16 servings

Ingredients	Directions
¾ cup raw hazelnuts, skin removed	*1* Pulse ½ cup of the hazelnuts in a food processor until they form ¾ cup of fine meal. Chop the remaining whole hazelnuts into small pieces and reserve.
5 tablespoons Homemade Chocolate Hazelnut Spread	
1 tablespoon coconut oil, melted	*2* In a large bowl, mix the hazelnut meal, chocolate hazelnut spread, coconut oil, vanilla, cacao powder, flaxseed meal, maple syrup, and salt. (I like using gloves and mixing by hand.)
2 teaspoons vanilla extract	
2 tablespoons raw cacao powder	*3* Make sixteen 1-inch truffles and roll each in the reserved chopped hazelnuts. Refrigerate for 20 minutes.
1 tablespoon flaxseed meal	
1 tablespoon maple syrup	
Pinch of salt	*4* Melt the chocolate chips and cacao butter slowly in a bowl over simmering water (double boiler).
¼ cup Paleo-friendly dark chocolate chips	
1 tablespoon cacao butter	*5* Using a fork, dip each truffle in the melted chocolate and set it on a baking sheet lined with parchment paper. Refrigerate until the chocolate hardens. Keep refrigerated.

Tip: To remove the skin from hazelnuts, you need to roast the nuts for a few minutes in the oven at 350 degrees, until the skin begins to crack. Then you can easily peel the skin off the nuts. Alternatively, you can purchase blanched hazelnuts, which are already skinned, to make the process much easier and faster.

Tip: Refrigerate your chocolate hazelnut spread until it's firm before making your truffles. You can replace the cacao butter in Step 4 with melted coconut oil.

Tip: If you enjoy Ferrero Rocher candies, consider this recipe your new go-to indulgence.

Per serving: Calories 107 (From Fat 81); Fat 9g (Saturated 2g); Cholesterol 0mg; Sodium 12mg; Carbohydrate 6g (Dietary Fiber 2g); Protein 2g.

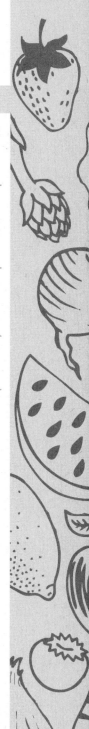

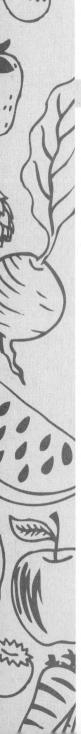

No-bake Double Chocolate Cookie Dough Bites

Prep time: 15 min, plus freezing time • **Yield:** 15 servings

Ingredients	Directions
¾ cup blanched almond flour	*1* Mix the almond flour, cacao powder, and shredded coconut in a bowl.
3 tablespoons raw cacao powder	
2 tablespoons unsweetened shredded coconut	*2* In a separate bowl, whisk the coconut oil, coconut milk, honey, vanilla, and 3 tablespoons of the chocolate chips.
3 tablespoons coconut oil, melted	
2 tablespoons full-fat coconut milk	*3* Using a rubber spatula, gently combine the wet ingredients and dry ingredients. Don't overmix.
4 tablespoons raw honey	*4* Freeze the dough for about 20 minutes.
1 teaspoon vanilla extract	
3 tablespoons Paleo-friendly mini chocolate chips, plus more for (optional) garnish	*5* Roll the chilled dough into 15 balls and then roll each in more chocolate chips (if desired).

Per serving: Calories 105 (From Fat 69); Fat 8g (Saturated 4g); Cholesterol 0mg; Sodium 3mg; Carbohydrate 8g (Dietary Fiber 1g); Protein 2g.

Honey-Roasted Cashew Drops

Prep time: 25 min • **Cook time:** 10 min • **Yield:** 20 servings

Ingredients	Directions
¼ cup **Paleo-friendly 70-percent dark chocolate, chopped**	**1** Preheat the oven to 300 degrees. Slowly melt the chocolate in a bowl over simmering water (double boiler). Add 1 tablespoon of the coconut oil and stir until smooth.
1 tablespoon plus 2 teaspoons coconut oil, melted and divided	**2** Heat the honey and the remaining coconut oil in a saucepan over medium heat. Mix in the cashews and stir to coat them.
1 tablespoon raw honey	
1 cup raw cashews	**3** Transfer the cashews to a baking sheet lined with parchment paper and roast in the oven for 10 minutes or until they start to turn golden-brown. Keep a close eye on them so they don't burn.
	4 Using a spoon, dip three or four cashews at a time in the melted chocolate and then place them on a sheet lined with parchment paper. Refrigerate the cashews until the chocolate hardens. Keep refrigerated.

Vary It! For a different slant, you can also toss the nuts into the chocolate and then spread the mixture on a sheet pan. Refrigerate til set, and break apart like brittle.

Per serving: Calories 55 (From Fat 38); Fat 4g (Saturated 2g); Cholesterol 0mg; Sodium 1mg; Carbohydrate 4g (Dietary Fiber 0g); Protein 1g.

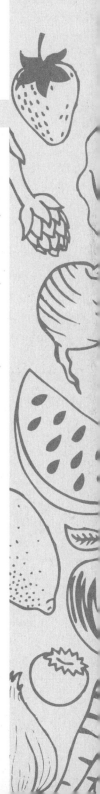

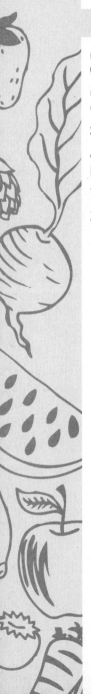

Dark Chocolate Orange Bonbons

Prep time: 25 min, plus chilling time • **Cook time:** 2 hr, 5 min • **Yield:** 15 servings

Ingredients	*Directions*
Chocolate Shell Coating (see the following recipe) **One 13.5-ounce can full-fat coconut milk** **3 tablespoons raw honey** **4 tablespoons raw cacao powder** **½ teaspoon vanilla extract** **Zest of 1 orange**	**1** Bring the coconut milk and honey to a boil over medium heat and simmer it over very low heat for about 2 hours, stirring occasionally. After 2 hours, the mixture should've thickened to have the consistency of sweetened condensed milk and not run off the spoon easily.
	2 Add the cacao powder and vanilla and cook for about 5 minutes, stirring constantly so the mixture doesn't burn. When the mixture starts to release off the bottom of the pan and has a very thick consistency, remove it from the stove.
	3 Add the orange zest and let the mixture cool to room temperature. Chill the cooled mixture in the fridge for about 2 hours.
	4 Grease your hands with butter and start rolling the chilled cacao mixture into balls, about 2 teaspoons per ball. Refrigerate the formed truffles while making the Chocolate Shell Coating.
	5 Dip each truffle in the Chocolate Shell Coating and then refrigerate on a sheet lined with parchment paper. Keep refrigerated.

Chocolate Shell Coating

2½ tablespoons cacao butter	*1* Melt the cacao butter in a bowl over simmering water (double boiler) until it reaches 122 degrees.
3½ tablespoons raw cacao powder	
1 tablespoons raw honey	*2* Add the remaining ingredients and mix until all are combined and the mixture reaches 122 degrees.
¼ teaspoon vanilla extract	

Per serving: Calories 110 (From Fat 79); Fat 9g (Saturated 7g); Cholesterol 0mg; Sodium 8mg; Carbohydrate 7g (Dietary Fiber 1g); Protein 1g.

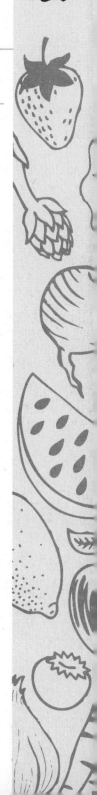

Coconut Truffles

Prep time: 15 min, plus chilling time • **Cook time:** 2 hrs for cooking; 2 hrs for cooling • **Yield:** 20 servings

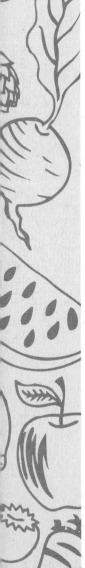

Ingredients	Directions
One 13.5-ounce can full-fat coconut milk	**1** Bring the coconut milk and honey to a boil over medium heat and simmer it over very low heat for about 2 hours, stirring occasionally. After 1½ to 2 hours, the mixture should've thickened to have the consistency of sweetened condensed milk and not run off the spoon easily.
3 tablespoons raw honey	
½ cup unsweetened shredded coconut, plus more for garnishing	
1 tablespoon pastured butter	**2** Add the shredded coconut, butter, and vanilla and cook for about 5 minutes, stirring frequently so it doesn't burn, about 10 minutes.
½ teaspoon vanilla extract	
	3 When the mixture starts to release off the bottom of the pan and has a very thick consistency, remove it from the stove and let it cool to room temperature. Chill the cooled mixture in the fridge for about 2 hours.
	4 Grease your hands with butter and roll the chilled mixture into 20 1-inch balls.
	5 Roll each truffle in shredded coconut. Store in the refrigerator.

Per serving: Calories 65 (From Fat 49); Fat 5g (Saturated 5g); Cholesterol 2mg; Sodium 6mg; Carbohydrate 4g (Dietary Fiber 0g); Protein 0g.

Macadamia-Caramel Clusters

Prep time: 20 min, plus freezing time • **Yield:** 9 servings

Ingredients	*Directions*
5 large Medjool dates, pitted	*1* In a blender or food processor, process the dates with the coconut milk, almond butter, and honey until creamy and smooth.
2 tablespoons full-fat coconut milk	
1 tablespoon almond butter	*2* Fold in the macadamia nuts, using a spoon.
½ tablespoon raw honey	
½ cup macadamia nuts, coarsely chopped	*3* Drop mixture by the tablespoonful onto a cookie sheet lined with parchment paper and freeze for 20 minutes.
4 ounces Paleo-friendly dark chocolate	
	4 Melt the chocolate in a bowl over simmering water (double boiler).
	5 Dip each cluster in the melted chocolate and set it back on the parchment paper. Refrigerate until the chocolate sets.

VaryIt! You can substitute the 84-Percent Dark Chocolate Sweetened with Honey earlier in this chapter for the dark chocolate in this recipe.

Per serving: Calories 251 (From Fat 158); Fat 18g (Saturated 6g); Cholesterol 0mg; Sodium 12mg; Carbohydrate 27g (Dietary Fiber 5g); Protein 3g.

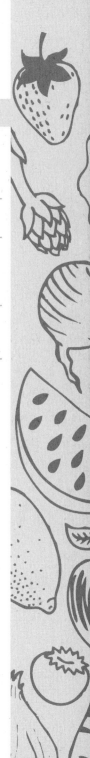

Chapter 8

Cookies

In This Chapter

▶ Enjoying cookies while living Paleo
▶ Whipping up healthy, tasty cookies

Having a warm chocolate chip cookie right out of the oven is the one thing I missed the most when I first started living Paleo. In the beginning of my Paleo journey, I decided not to eat any sweets at all, based on the conventional wisdom that all sweets are equally bad. I was still learning about the principles of the diet and how each ingredient affected my health. The restrictions I put on myself set me back many times, especially when I walked by my favorite cookie shop and couldn't resist eating a cookie (or three) to satisfy my cravings. At that point, I didn't know that I could tinker with the ingredients to make a healthier cookie.

Depriving yourself cold-turkey of foods your body is so used to eating doesn't work well in most cases. That's why I'm excited to share with you some of my favorite cookie recipes. I hope the recipes in this chapter make living Paleo easier and more enjoyable. Soon, you'll no longer crave sweet foods as much. You'll find that having a cookie now and then is quite a treat and very satisfying.

All the cookie recipes in this chapter follow Paleo nutritional guidelines and contain no grains, gluten, soy, or other processed ingredients. These recipes also follow fundamental cookie rules: They taste delicious and burst with flavor! So flip through the following pages, grab a pen and paper for making a shopping list, and begin experimenting with the wonderful selection of cookie recipes in this chapter.

Dulce de Leche Cashew Cookies

Prep time: 30 min, plus chilling time • **Cook time:** 25 min • **Yield:** 10 servings

Ingredients	Directions
Dulce de Leche (see the following recipe)	**1** Preheat the oven to 350 degrees. Line a baking sheet with parchment paper.
¾ cup raw cashews, divided	
½ cup blanched almond flour	**2** Using a food processor, pulse ½ cup of the cashews until you get a flourlike consistency. Coarsely chop the remaining ¼ cup of the cashews and set aside.
2 tablespoons organic coconut palm sugar	
1 teaspoon arrowroot powder	**3** Mix the almond flour, coconut sugar, arrowroot powder, and salt with the processed cashews until combined.
¼ teaspoon salt	
1 egg	**4** In a separate bowl, beat the egg, butter, and vanilla with a handheld or electric mixer.
5 tablespoons unsalted pastured butter, softened	
½ teaspoon vanilla extract	**5** Mix the wet ingredients and dry ingredients, using a rubber spatula. Freeze the dough for 20 minutes.
	6 Roll the chilled dough into balls — about 1½ tablespoons of dough per ball. Roll each ball in the reserved chopped cashews.
	7 Using your thumb or the back of a teaspoon, make a depression in the center of each ball.
	8 Bake the cookies until the bottoms and edges start to turn brown, approximately 15 minutes. Immediately after you remove the cookies from the oven, press the center of each cookie again. (Don't use your thumb this time; they'll be hot.)
	9 Allow the cookies to cool on a wire rack. Fill each cookie with the Dulce de Leche and serve. Store in an airtight container in the fridge.

Dulce de Leche

2 tablespoons water

¼ cup organic coconut palm sugar

½ cup full-fat coconut milk

1 teaspoon vanilla extract

Pinch of salt

1 Bring the water and coconut palm sugar to a boil over medium heat, stirring the mixture constantly.

2 Add the remaining ingredients and cook for about 10 minutes over medium heat, stirring constantly so that it doesn't burn. The mixture will start to thicken and turn darker.

3 Allow the mixture to cool and then refrigerate it for 30 minutes.

Per serving: *Calories 194 (From Fat 132); Fat 15g (Saturated 6g); Cholesterol 34mg; Sodium 90mg; Carbohydrate 13g (Dietary Fiber 1g); Protein 4g.*

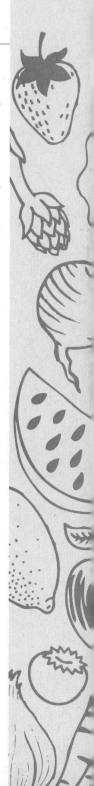

Chocolate Sandwich Cookies with Cookie Dough Filling

Prep time: 40 min, plus freezing time • **Cook time:** 10–12 min • **Yield:** 13 servings

Ingredients	Directions
Cookie Dough Filling (see the following recipe)	*1* Preheat the oven to 350 degrees. Melt the chocolate chips in a bowl over simmering water (double boiler); remove the bowl from the heat and whisk in the coconut oil, vanilla extract, and egg.
⅓ cup Paleo-friendly dark chocolate chips	
⅓ cup coconut oil, melted	
½ teaspoon vanilla extract	*2* In a separate bowl, mix the almond flour, cacao powder, baking soda, and salt.
1 room temperature egg	
1 cup blanched almond flour	*3* Using a rubber spatula, mix the wet ingredients and dry ingredients gently until just combined. Cover the dough and freeze for about 15 minutes.
⅓ cup raw cacao powder	
¼ teaspoon baking soda	*4* Using a rolling pin, roll the chilled dough between two sheets of parchment paper to ¼-inch thickness.
⅛ teaspoon salt	
	5 Cut cookies with a round 2-inch cookie cutter. If the dough gets sticky or is hard to work with, return it to the freezer for another 10 to 15 minutes as needed.
	6 Bake the cookies on a cookie sheet lined with parchment paper for 10 to 12 minutes. Let the cookies cool on the baking sheet for 5 minutes and then transfer them to a wire rack.
	7 Roll the Cookie Dough Filling into small balls, about 2 teaspoons of dough per cookie. Gently press each dough ball between two cookies. Store in an airtight container in the fridge.

Cookie Dough Filling

3 tablespoons coconut oil, melted

1 tablespoon raw honey

1 teaspoon vanilla extract

¾ cup blanched almond flour

¼ cup Paleo-friendly dark chocolate chips

1 In a large bowl, whisk the coconut oil, honey, and vanilla.

2 Add the remaining ingredients and gently mix by hand. Don't overmix the dough, or it will get oily.

Per serving: Calories 237 (From Fat 192); Fat 21g (Saturated 11g); Cholesterol 14mg; Sodium 58mg; Carbohydrate 11g (Dietary Fiber 4g); Protein 5g.

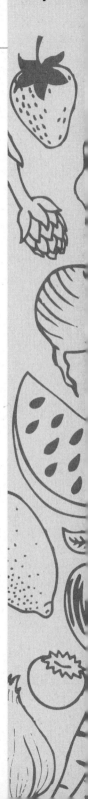

Banana Cinnamon Cookies

Prep time: 20 min • **Cook time:** 10–15 min • **Yield:** 17 servings

Ingredients	Directions
1½ cups blanched almond flour	**1** Preheat the oven to 350 degrees and line a cookie sheet with parchment paper. In a large bowl, mix the almond flour, flaxseed meal, cinnamon, coconut sugar, baking soda, and salt.
2 tablespoons flaxseed meal	
½ teaspoon ground cinnamon	
2 tablespoons organic coconut palm sugar	**2** Process the bananas, coconut oil, vanilla, and egg in a food processor until the bananas are pureed and all ingredients are combined. Add the mixture to the bowl with the dry ingredients and gently mix with a rubber spatula to combine ingredients.
½ teaspoon baking soda	
Pinch of salt	
½ to ¾ cup chopped bananas	**3** Stir in the macadamia nuts (if desired). Using a medium cookie scoop, scoop the batter onto a cookie sheet lined with parchment paper. Flatten each cookie slightly with your hand. If the batter sticks to your hands, wet them with water.
¼ cup coconut oil, melted	
2 teaspoon vanilla extract	
1 room temperature egg	
¼ cup macadamia nuts, chopped (optional)	**4** Bake the cookies for about 10 to 15 minutes or until the edges and bottoms start to brown or a toothpick inserted into the center comes out clean. Let the cookies cool on a wire rack.

Tip: If you don't have a medium-sized cookie scoop, use about 1½ tablespoons of dough per cookie.

Vary It! You can punch up these cookies with a chocolate coating. Melt 4 tablespoons of Paleo-friendly chocolate chips in a double boiler. Dip the bottom of each cookie in the melted chocolate, put them back on the cooled, parchment-lined cookie sheet, and refrigerate them until the chocolate hardens.

Per serving: Calories 107 (From Fat 77); Fat 9g (Saturated 3g); Cholesterol 11mg; Sodium 54mg; Carbohydrate 6g (Dietary Fiber 2g); Protein 3g.

Chocolate Chip Zucchini Cookies

Prep time: 20 min • **Cook time:** 12 min • **Yield:** 17 servings

Ingredients	*Directions*
1½ cups blanched almond flour	**1** Preheat the oven to 325 degrees. In a large bowl, mix the almond flour, baking soda, coconut sugar, cacao powder, and salt.
½ teaspoon baking soda	
3 to 4 tablespoons organic coconut palm sugar	
¼ cup raw cacao powder	**2** In a separate bowl, whisk the egg, coconut milk, coconut oil, and vanilla; then stir in the zucchini.
Pinch of salt	
¾ cup finely grated and chopped zucchini	**3** Combine the wet and dry ingredients and mix gently with rubber spatula to form a dough. Don't overmix, or the dough will become oily.
1 large room temperature egg	
2 tablespoons full-fat coconut milk	**4** Fold in the chocolate chips and macadamia nuts (if desired).
4 tablespoons coconut oil, melted	**5** Scoop the dough, about 1½ tablespoons per cookie, onto a baking sheet lined with parchment paper. Bake until a toothpick inserted into the center comes out clean, approximately 12 minutes.
1 teaspoon vanilla extract	
⅓ cup Paleo-friendly chocolate chips	
¼ cup macadamia nuts, chopped (optional)	**6** Place the baking sheet on a wire rack and allow the cookies to cool.

Per serving: Calories 135 (From Fat 96); Fat 11g (Saturated 5g); Cholesterol 11mg; Sodium 55mg; Carbohydrate 8g (Dietary Fiber 2g); Protein 3g.

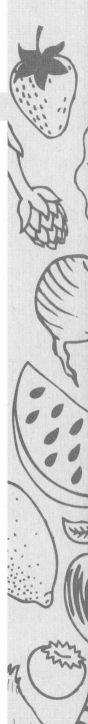

No-bake Chocolate Cookies

Prep time: 15 min • **Yield:** 20 servings

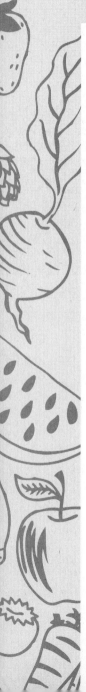

Ingredients	Directions
2½ tablespoons cacao butter	**1** Melt the cacao butter and chocolate chips in bowl over simmering water (double boiler).
⅓ cup Paleo-friendly chocolate chips	
3½ tablespoons raw cacao powder	**2** Whisk in the cacao powder, coconut oil, honey, and almond butter.
1 tablespoon coconut oil, melted	**3** Add the pecans and shredded coconut and mix to combine.
1 tablespoon raw honey	
4 tablespoons almond butter	**4** Scoop the mixture by tablespoonful onto a cookie sheet lined with parchment paper. Flatten cookies slightly with your hand and refrigerate until the cookies harden.
½ cup pecans, chopped	
½ cup unsweetened shredded coconut	

Vary It! You can replace the cacao butter in Step 1 with melted coconut oil.

Per serving: Calories 104 (From Fat 82); Fat 9g (Saturated 4g); Cholesterol 0mg; Sodium 9mg; Carbohydrate 5g (Dietary Fiber 1g); Protein 2g.

Flourless Chocolate Chip Cookies

Prep time: 20 min • **Cook time:** 15 min • **Yield:** 18 servings

Ingredients	Directions
1 cup almonds **1 cup pecans** **1 large room temperature egg** **½ teaspoon vanilla extract** **3 tablespoons raw honey** **⅓ cup Paleo-friendly chocolate chips, divided** **Pinch of salt**	*1* Preheat the oven to 350 degrees. Process the almonds and pecans in a food processor until they're creamy and smooth, scraping the sides as needed.
	2 In a large bowl, whisk the egg, vanilla, honey, and salt and then gently fold in the almond/pecan butter and chocolate chips, reserving a couple of tablespoons of the chips for topping the cookies.
	3 Spoon tablespoonfuls of the batter onto a cookie sheet lined with parchment paper.
	4 Top each cookie with a few of the reserved chocolate chips and bake for about 15 minutes or until the edges and top start to turn brown.
	5 Let the cookies cool on a wire rack.

Per serving: *Calories 116 (From Fat 83); Fat 9g (Saturated 1g); Cholesterol 10mg; Sodium 12mg; Carbohydrate 7g (Dietary Fiber 2g); Protein 3g.*

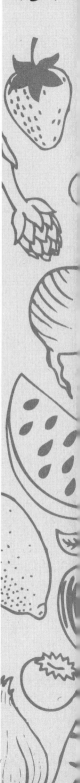

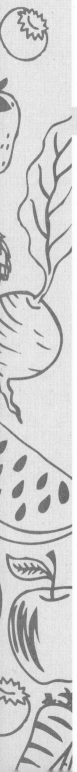

Almond Cookies with Chocolate Avocado Fudge Frosting

Prep time: 30 min, plus chilling time • **Cook time:** 17 min • **Yield:** 22 servings

Ingredients	Directions
Chocolate Avocado Fudge Frosting (see the following recipe)	**1** Preheat the oven to 325 degrees. In a large bowl, combine the almond flour, coconut sugar, baking soda, and salt.
1½ cups blanched almond flour	
3 tablespoons organic coconut palm sugar	**2** In a separate bowl, whisk the coconut milk, coconut oil, vanilla, and egg. Combine the wet ingredients and dry ingredients and gently mix with a rubber spatula. Refrigerate the dough for 30 minutes.
½ teaspoon baking soda	
Pinch of salt	
2½ tablespoons full-fat coconut milk	**3** Spoon ½ tablespoon-size balls of the chilled dough onto a cookie sheet lined with parchment paper and then press each with the palm of your hand to flatten.
¼ cup coconut oil, melted	
1 teaspoon vanilla extract	**4** Bake for 17 minutes or until the edges start to turn golden brown.
1 room temperature egg	
	5 Set the baking sheet on a wire rack and let the cookies cool. Top each cookie with the Chocolate Avocado Fudge Frosting and serve.

Chocolate Avocado Fudge Frosting

2 tablespoons cacao butter

6 tablespoons raw cacao powder

3 tablespoons raw honey

1 teaspoon vanilla extract

1 cup mashed avocado

1 Melt the cacao butter in a bowl over simmering water (double boiler).

2 Remove the bowl from the heat and mix in the cacao powder, honey, and vanilla.

3 In a blender or food processor, pulse the chocolate mixture and avocado until creamy. You can adjust the sweetness of the frosting to your liking by adding more honey. Store frosting in the fridge for up to 1 week.

Tip: I recommend using Haas avocados for this frosting. You'll need about 2 small Haas avocados to get the 1 cup of avocado called for.

Per serving: Calories 120 (From Fat 96); Fat 10g (Saturated 4g); Cholesterol 9mg; Sodium 44mg; Carbohydrate 7g (Dietary Fiber 2g); Protein 3g.

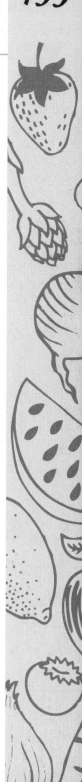

Honey Graham Crackers

Prep time: 35 min, plus freezing time • **Cook time:** 9–11 min • **Yield:** 20 servings

Ingredients	Directions
¾ cup blanched almond four	**1** Preheat the oven to 350 degrees. Mix the almond flour, flaxseed meal, arrowroot powder, baking soda, and salt in a bowl.
2 tablespoons flaxseed meal	
⅓ cup arrowroot powder	
¼ teaspoon baking soda	**2** In a separate bowl, whisk the butter, coconut milk, vanilla, and honey.
Pinch of salt	
2½ tablespoons pastured butter, softened	**3** Gently mix the dry ingredients and wet ingredients together using a rubber spatula.
1 tablespoon full-fat coconut milk	**4** Place the dough between two sheets of parchment paper and roll it to ⅛-inch thickness with a rolling pin and then freeze for 15 to 20 minutes.
2 teaspoons vanilla extract	
2 tablespoons raw honey	**5** Cut the dough into 3-inch squares with a knife or pizza cutter and place each square on a baking sheet lined with parchment paper. If the dough is too soft to work with, freeze it for 20 minutes.
	6 Bake at 350 degrees for 9 to 11 minutes or until lightly golden. Let the crackers cool on the baking sheet set over a wire rack.

Marshmallow

5 tablespoons water, divided

1 teaspoon grass-fed gelatin

⅓ cup raw honey

¼ teaspoon vanilla extract

pinch of salt

egg white from 1 small egg

3 ounces Paleo-friendly 70-percent dark chocolate

1 In a large bowl mix the gelatin with 2½ tablespoons of water (reserve remaining water). While the gelatin is dissolving, add the other half of the water to a saucepan and mix in the honey and salt.

2 Place a candy thermometer in the saucepan and heat the mixture slowly, stirring constantly until it reaches 240°F. When the mixture reaches this temperature, immediately remove from the heat.

3 Using a stand or hand mixer slowly add the honey to the dissolved gelatin and whip until it becomes thick, like marshmallow cream.

4 In a separate bowl, whip the egg white until it forms soft peaks; then add the vanilla and marshmallow cream, and continue to whip to combine ingredients.

5 Transfer marshmallow to a 7x5-inch dish lined with parchment paper. Let marshmallow set in the fridge then cut into squares.

6 To make s'mores, place a piece of dark chocolate and the marshmallow between two crackers.

Per serving: Calories 76 (From Fat 47); Fat 5g (Saturated 2g); Cholesterol 5mg; Sodium 33mg; Carbohydrate 6g (Dietary Fiber 1g); Protein 1g.

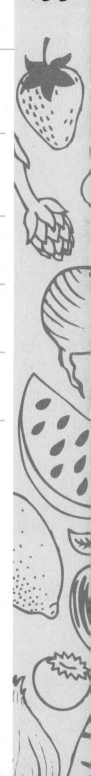

Soft and Chewy Chocolate Chip Cookies

Prep time: 15 min, plus chilling time • **Cook time:** 8–10 min • **Yield:** 10 servings

Ingredients	Directions
1 cup blanched almond flour	**1** Preheat the oven to 350 degrees. In a medium bowl, mix the almond flour, arrowroot powder, and baking soda.
1 tablespoon arrowroot powder	
½ teaspoon baking soda	**2** In a separate bowl, beat the butter with an electric mixer and then mix in the egg, vanilla, and honey.
4 tablespoons room temperature pastured butter	
1 egg	**3** Combine the wet ingredients and dry ingredients and mix gently with a rubber spatula until combined. Stir in the chocolate chips.
1 teaspoon vanilla extract	
1 tablespoon raw honey	**4** Refrigerate the dough for about 15 minutes.
⅓ cup Paleo-friendly chocolate chips	**5** Scoop the dough by tablespoonfuls onto a baking sheet lined with parchment paper and then flatten each cookie with the palm of your hand. The cookies should be about 2 inches apart.
	6 Bake until the cookies are golden around the edges but still soft in the center, about 8 to 10 minutes.
	7 Remove the cookies from the oven; let them cool on the baking sheet for 1 to 2 minutes and then slide the parchment paper off the baking sheet and onto a wire rack to cool completely.

Per serving: Calories 154 (From Fat 113); Fat 13g (Saturated 5g); Cholesterol 31mg; Sodium 75mg; Carbohydrate 9g (Dietary Fiber 5g); Protein 4g.

Coconut Chocolate Chip Cookies

Prep time: 15 min • **Cook time:** 10 min • **Yield:** 20 servings

Ingredients	Directions
1 room temperature egg	**1** Preheat the oven to 350 degrees. In a large bowl, whisk the egg slightly.
½ cup coconut butter, melted	
½ cup organic coconut palm sugar	**2** Add the coconut butter, coconut sugar, shredded coconut, salt, baking soda, lemon zest, and vanilla. Mix with a rubber spatula until combined. Fold in the chocolate chips, reserving a couple of tablespoons of the chips for topping the cookies.
½ cup unsweetened shredded coconut	
⅛ teaspoon salt	
½ teaspoon baking soda	**3** Line a baking sheet with parchment paper and scoop ½-tablespoon-size pieces of dough onto the paper, spacing the cookies 2 inches apart.
2 teaspoons lemon zest	
½ teaspoon vanilla extract	
⅓ cup Paleo-friendly dark chocolate chips , plus more for topping	**4** Top each cookie with two or three of the reserved chocolate chips.
	5 Bake for 10 minutes or until the edges and bottoms start to turn brown.
	6 Allow the cookies to cool on a wire rack.

Tip: To melt coconut butter in the jar, place the jar in a large saucepan with simmering water. You can save some money by making your own coconut butter. Blend 2 cups of unsweetened shredded coconut in a high-speed blender or a food processor until creamy, scraping the sides as needed.

Per serving: Calories 97 (From Fat 62); Fat 7g (Saturated 6g); Cholesterol 9mg; Sodium 55mg; Carbohydrate 10g (Dietary Fiber 2g); Protein 1g.

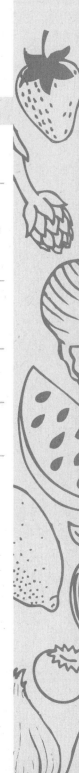

Chocolate Hazelnut Cream-Filled Chocolate Chip Cookies

Prep time: 25 min, plus overnight • **Cook time:** 10–12 min • **Yield:** 13 servings

Ingredients	Directions
Homemade Chocolate Hazelnut Spread	**1** Chill the Homemade Chocolate Hazelnut Spread in the refrigerator overnight or until it hardens.
1½ cups blanched almond flour	
¼ cup raw cacao powder	**2** Preheat the oven to 350 degrees. In a large bowl, mix the almond flour, cacao powder, coconut sugar, baking soda, and salt.
4 tablespoons organic coconut palm sugar	
1 teaspoon baking soda	**3** In a separate bowl, whisk the coconut milk, coconut oil, vanilla, and egg.
¼ teaspoon salt	
3 tablespoons full-fat coconut milk	**4** Using a rubber spatula, mix the dry ingredients and wet ingredients together. Don't overmix.
4 tablespoons coconut oil, melted	**5** Gently fold in the chocolate chips, reserving a couple of tablespoons of the chips for topping the cookies. Cover the bowl and freeze for 30 minutes.
1 teaspoon vanilla extract	
1 room temperature egg	
¼ cup Paleo-friendly dark chocolate chips, divided	**6** Scoop about 1½ tablespoon-size pieces of the chilled dough onto a baking sheet lined with parchment paper. Using your thumb, make an indentation in the center of each ball large enough to fit 1 teaspoon of chocolate hazelnut spread.
	7 Add 1 teaspoon of the chilled spread in the center of each cookie, then wrap and press the cookie dough around it to cover the filling entirely.
	8 Roll each cookie into a ball and then gently press down to flatten, being careful not to split them open. If your dough or spread softens and becomes hard to work with, chill it for a few minutes.

9 Top the cookies with a few of the reserved chocolate chips and bake for approximately 10 to 12 minutes.

10 Allow the cookies to cool on the baking sheet for 5 minutes; then move them to a wire rack.

Tip: You can find the recipe for Homemade Chocolate Hazelnut Spread in Chapter 11.

Per serving: Calories 194 (From Fat 141); Fat 16g (Saturated 7g); Cholesterol 14mg; Sodium 157mg; Carbohydrate 12g (Dietary Fiber 3g); Protein 5g.

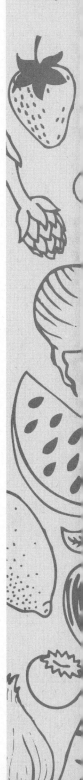

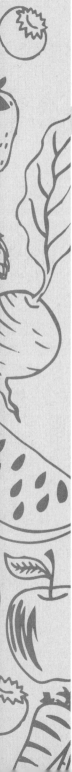

Chocolate-Strawberry Cookie Sandwiches

Prep time: 25 min, plus chilling time • **Cook time:** 15 min • **Yield:** 9 servings

Ingredients	Directions
½ cup plus 6 tablespoons blanched almond flour	*1* Preheat the oven to 325 degrees. Mix the almond flour and arrowroot powder in a bowl.
¼ cup arrowroot powder	
½ cup Paleo-friendly chocolate chips, divided	*2* Melt ¼ cup of the chocolate chips in a double boiler and reserve the remaining ¼ cup. When the chocolate is melted, remove it from the stove and stir in the vanilla and coconut oil until smooth.
2 teaspoons vanilla extract	
3 tablespoons coconut oil, melted	*3* Gently mix the dry ingredients into the wet ingredients using a rubber spatula.
6 tablespoons Sugar-Free Strawberry Jam	
1 tablespoon cacao butter	*4* Roll the chilled dough between two sheets of parchment paper until it's ⅛-inch to ¼-inch thick and refrigerate for 30 minutes.
	5 Cut the cookies with a 2-inch cookie cutter and then place them on a large baking sheet lined with parchment paper. Bake for approximately 15 minutes and allow the cookies to cool on a wire rack.
	6 Add 2 teaspoons of the Sugar-Free Strawberry Jam to the center of nine of the cookies. Top with the remaining nine cookies and press down to spread the jam between the two cookies.

7 Melt the reserved ¼ cup of chocolate chips and the cacao butter in a bowl over simmering water (double boiler). Gently spread the mixture over the top of each cookie. Keep refrigerated in an airtight container.

Tip: Look for the Sugar-Free Strawberry Jam recipe in Chapter 11.

Vary It! You can replace the cacao butter in Step 7 with melted coconut oil.

Per serving: Calories 178 (From Fat 121); Fat 13g (Saturated 8g); Cholesterol 0mg; Sodium 3mg; Carbohydrate 13g (Dietary Fiber 2g); Protein 2g.

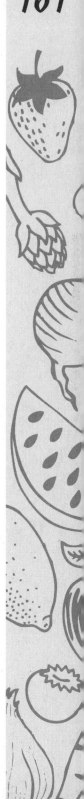

Macadamia Thumbprint Cookies with Chocolate Filling

Prep time: 25 min, plus overnight • **Cook time:** 8–10 min • **Yield:** 10 servings

Ingredients	Directions
Chocolate Filling (see the following recipe)	*1* Preheat the oven at 350 degrees and line a baking sheet with parchment paper.
⅓ cup raw macadamia nuts, chopped	*2* In a bowl, mix the macadamia nuts, almond flour, coconut oil, honey, and salt. Refrigerate the dough for 30 minutes.
¾ cup blanched almond flour	
3 tablespoons coconut oil, melted	*3* Shape the chilled dough into 1-inch balls and press your thumb into the center, creating an indentation.
1 tablespoon raw honey	*4* Fill each cookie with 1 teaspoon of the Chocolate Filling.
Pinch of salt	
	5 Bake the cookies until the bottoms and edges start to turn brown, approximately 8 to 10 minutes.
	6 Let the cookies cool on the baking sheet over a wire rack.

Chocolate Filling

2½ tablespoons cacao butter

3½ tablespoons cacao paste

¼ teaspoon vanilla extract

1¼ tablespoons coconut cream

1 tablespoon raw honey

1 Melt the cacao butter and cacao paste in a bowl over simmering water (double boiler).

2 Remove the bowl from the heat and stir in the vanilla, honey, and coconut cream until smooth.

Tip: Coconut cream is the thick cream that forms on the top of a can of full-fat coconut milk when you leave it in the fridge overnight, discarding the water.

Vary It! You can replace the cacao paste in the filling with 100-percent unsweetened dark chocolate.

Per serving: Calories 269 (From Fat 231); Fat 26g (Saturated 12g); Cholesterol 29mg; Sodium 29mg; Carbohydrate 8g (Dietary Fiber 2g); Protein 4g.

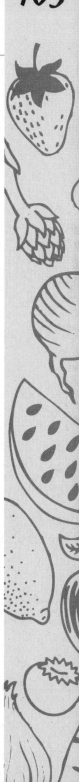

Soft and Chewy Butter Cookies

Prep time: 15 min • **Cook time:** 10 min • **Yield:** 10 servings

Ingredients	Directions
4 tablespoons room temperature pastured butter	*1* Preheat the oven to 350 degrees. Using an electric handheld or stand mixer, cream the butter and coconut sugar.
2 tablespoons organic coconut palm sugar	
2 egg whites	*2* Add the egg whites and then the vanilla extract and continue beating.
2 teaspoons vanilla extract	
½ cup blanched almond flour	*3* Using a rubber spatula, mix in the almond flour until all ingredients are combined (the dough will be soft).
70-percent dark chocolate, chopped (optional)	
	4 Spoon ½-tablespoon-size pieces of dough onto a baking sheet lined with parchment paper, spacing them 2 inches apart and giving them room to spread while baking.
	5 Bake for 10 minutes or until light golden brown around the edges. Let the cookies cool on the baking sheet over a wire rack.
	6 Melt the dark chocolate in a bowl over simmering water (double boiler) and drizzle on top of the cooled cookies (optional).

Note: These are thin cookies, and they spread while baking.

Per serving: Calories 106 (From Fat 77); Fat 9g (Saturated 4g); Cholesterol 12mg; Sodium 15mg; Carbohydrate 6g (Dietary Fiber 1g); Protein 2g.

Crunchy Chocolate Almond Cookies

Prep time: 20 min • **Cook time:** 10 min • **Yield:** 15 servings

Ingredients	Directions
½ cup plus 6 tablespoons blanched almond flour ¼ cup arrowroot powder	*1* Preheat the oven to 350 degrees and line a baking sheet with parchment paper. In a medium bowl, mix the almond flour and arrowroot powder.
¼ cup Paleo-friendly chocolate chips 1 tablespoon full-fat coconut milk	*2* Melt the chocolate chips in a bowl over simmering water (double boiler). Add the coconut milk, vanilla extract, and butter and mix until smooth.
½ tablespoon vanilla extract 4 tablespoons pastured butter	*3* Gently fold the almond flour mixture into the chocolate to make a soft biscuit dough.
15 almonds (optional)	*4* Spoon the dough into a piping bag fitted with a large star nozzle. Alternatively, you can use a zip-top bag and cut the tip off one corner.
	5 Pipe 15 cookies (about 2½ inches each) onto the baking sheet.
	6 Top each cookie with an almond in the center (if desired).
	7 Bake for 10 minutes or until the cookies are firm and starting to brown.
	8 Cool the cookies for about 10 minutes on the baking sheet and then lift them carefully onto a wire rack to cool completely. Store in an airtight container.

Per serving: Calories 96 (From Fat 70); Fat 8g (Saturated 3g); Cholesterol 8mg; Sodium 3mg; Carbohydrate 6g (Dietary Fiber 1g); Protein 2g.

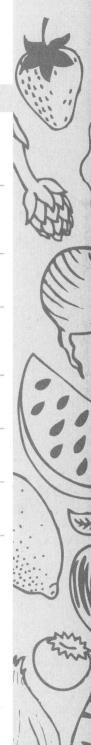

Pecan Cookie Sandwiches with Chocolate Filling

Prep time: 25 min • **Cook time:** 10 min • **Yield:** 10 servings

Ingredients	Directions
Chocolate Sandwich Filling (see the following recipe)	**1** Preheat the oven to 325 degrees and line a cookie sheet with parchment paper.
1 cup pecans	
4 tablespoons coconut flour	**2** In a food processor, pulse the pecans and coconut flour until they have a flourlike consistency. Pulse in the arrowroot powder, baking soda, and salt and then the honey, cream, coconut oil, and vanilla.
1 teaspoon arrowroot powder	
½ teaspoon baking soda	
Pinch of salt	
1½ tablespoons raw honey	**3** Roll the dough into a ball and press it between two sheets of parchment paper to ⅛-inch thickness.
1 tablespoon full-fat coconut milk	
5 tablespoons coconut oil, melted	**4** Cut the dough with a 2-inch round cookie cutter and then place cookies onto the prepared baking sheet.
½ teaspoon vanilla extract	
	5 Bake for about 10 minutes or until the edges start to turn brown.
	6 Let the cookies cool completely on a wire rack. Add about 1 tablespoon of the Chocolate Sandwich Filling to half of the cookies and top with the remaining cookies, pressing down to spread the chocolate around.

Chocolate Sandwich Filling

5 tablespoons cacao butter

7 tablespoons raw cacao powder

4 tablespoons raw honey

½ teaspoon vanilla extract

1 Melt the cacao butter in a bowl over simmering water (double boiler).

2 Mix in the remaining ingredients until all combined and smooth.

Vary It! You can replace the full-fat coconut milk in the cookie recipe with pastured heavy cream.

Per serving: Calories 269 (From Fat 206); Fat 23g (Saturated 13g); Cholesterol 2mg; Sodium 86mg; Carbohydrate 15g (Dietary Fiber 3g); Protein 2g.

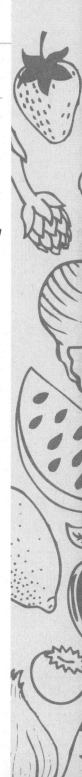

Chocolate Chip Cookie Sticks

Prep time: 15 min, plus freezing time • **Cook time:** 10–15 min • **Yield:** 25 servings

Ingredients	Directions
1½ cups blanched almond flour	*1* Preheat the oven to 325 degrees. In a bowl, mix the almond flour, coconut sugar, baking soda, and salt.
3 to 4 tablespoons organic coconut palm sugar	
½ teaspoon baking soda	*2* In a separate bowl, whisk the egg and then mix in the coconut milk, coconut oil, and vanilla.
Pinch of salt	
1 room temperature egg	*3* Gently mix the dry ingredients and wet ingredients using a rubber spatula, being careful not to overmix. Freeze the dough for 30 minutes.
2½ tablespoons full-fat coconut milk	
4 tablespoons coconut oil, melted	*4* Roll the chilled dough between two sheets of parchment paper into a 12-inch-x-6-inch rectangle about about ¼-inch thick.
1 teaspoon vanilla extract	
⅓ cup Paleo-friendly chocolate chips	*5* Sprinkle the top with the chocolate chips and bake for about 10 to 15 minutes or until the edges and top start to turn brown.
	6 Remove the sheet from the oven and immediately cut the cookie into 3-inch-x-1-inch sticks. Don't separate the pieces until the cookies have cooled.
	7 Set the pan on a wire rack to cool.

Per serving: Calories 82 (From Fat 60); Fat 7g (Saturated 3g); Cholesterol 7mg; Sodium 37mg; Carbohydrate 5g (Dietary Fiber 1g); Protein 2g.

Chapter 9

Ice Cream and Frozen Treats

Dairy is typically an essential ingredient for making ice cream because of its fat content, but it's also a somewhat controversial ingredient in Paleo circles (which I explain in a bit). However, almost all the ice cream recipes in this chapter are dairy-free. How is that possible? Well, they simply replace heavy cream with coconut milk, which is also very high in fat and helps make the ice cream creamy. Personally, I like using a combination of half coconut milk and half cream when making ice cream. You can take this approach for any of the recipes in this chapter; if you prefer, you can use cream only or coconut milk only.

Note: Dairy is a hot-button Paleo issue for a couple of reasons. Some argue that dairy wasn't part of our Paleolithic ancestors' diet or evolutionary heritage and that it's therefore part of the disease-causing problem. Others point to studies that show pasture-raised, grass-fed dairy as being a highly nutritious food with many health benefits, providing a rich source of both *conjugated linoleic acid* (a healthy fat known as CLA) and vitamin K2. CLA has been shown to have anti-cancer properties and lower the risk of heart attacks, while vitamin K2 promotes bone health and helps prevent atherosclerosis and cardiovascular disease.

Above all, Paleo isn't a restrictive diet. The main focus is to supply your body with essential nutrients and observe closely how your body responds to the foods you eat. Many people that have autoimmune problems and are lactose intolerant don't do well eating conventional dairy, but they often have no problems consuming high-fat, raw, unpasteurized dairy from grass-fed animals. The best thing to do is eliminate dairy completely for at least 30 days and then slowly reintroduce it to see how your body responds to it.

Fat choice aside, here are a couple of additional pointers for making Paleo ice cream that supports your health without leaving you feeling deprived:

✔ Use arrowroot powder, unflavored gelatin (from pastured animals), or guar gum. These ingredients prevent ice crystals from forming after you freeze the ice cream and preserve that lovely, creamy texture. They also provide a great way to make homemade ice cream without an ice cream machine, and omitting eggs when making the custard.

✔ If your body is sensitive to eating eggs, you can omit them in any of the ice cream recipes in this chapter.

Coffee Chocolate Chip Ice Cream

Prep time: 10 min, plus overnight • **Cook time:** 5 min • **Yield:** 1 quart

Ingredients	Directions
3 tablespoons organic ground coffee (or instant coffee)	**1** In a medium saucepan, whisk the coffee, coconut milk, arrowroot powder, egg, honey, and salt.
One 13.5-ounce can full-fat coconut milk	
2 tablespoons arrowroot powder	**2** Heat the mixture slowly over medium heat until it starts to bubble and thickens, stirring frequently. Let it cool for 5 minutes and then mix in the vanilla and refrigerate overnight.
1 egg	
2 tablespoons raw honey	**3** Stir the chocolate chips into the chilled mixture. Place the mixture in an ice cream maker and process it according to the manufacturer's instructions until it reaches a soft-serve consistency.
Pinch of salt	
2 teaspoons vanilla extract	
¼ cup Paleo-friendly chocolate chips	**4** Serve immediately or spoon the ice cream into an air-tight container and freeze until firm, about 2 hours.

Tip: You can substitute the 84-percent Dark Chocolate Sweetened with Honey from Chapter 7 for the chocolate chips in this recipe.

Per serving: Calories 159 (From Fat 109); Fat 12g (Saturated 9g); Cholesterol 23mg; Sodium 39mg; Carbohydrate 13g (Dietary Fiber 1g); Protein 2g.

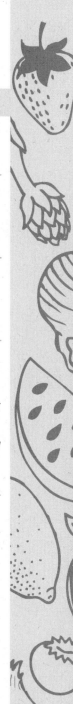

Pineapple Coconut Ice Cream

Prep time: 15 min, plus overnight • **Cook time:** 5 min • **Yield:** 1 quart

Ingredients	Directions
1½ cups unsweetened shredded coconut	**1** Blend the water and shredded coconut in a blender for 2 minutes. Strain the milk through a fine mesh strainer or cheesecloth into a medium saucepan (this process yields 2½ cups of coconut milk).
3 cups hot water	
2 tablespoons arrowroot powder	**2** Whisk in the arrowroot powder until dissolved. Mix in the egg, honey, and salt. Bring mixture to a light boil slowly over medium heat, stirring frequently. When it starts to bubble, remove it from the heat.
1 egg	
3 tablespoons raw honey	
Pinch of salt	**3** Let the mixture cool for 5 minutes and then mix in the vanilla and refrigerate overnight.
1 tablespoon vanilla extract	
1 cup diced fresh pineapple	
½ cup unsweetened dried coconut flakes	**4** Place the mixture in an ice cream maker and process it according to the manufacturer's instructions until it reaches a soft-serve consistency.
	5 Mix the chopped pineapple and coconut flakes into the chilled ice cream.
	6 Serve immediately or spoon the ice cream into an air-tight container and freeze until firm, about 2 hours.

Tip: If you don't want to make your own coconut milk, you can skip Step 1 and start Step 2 by putting 2½ cups of full-fat canned coconut milk in a saucepan.

Tip: If you can find mature coconuts in your grocery store, consider substituting chopped fresh coconut meat in place of the flakes in Step 4. Mature coconuts have thicker meat than young coconuts, whose meat is very soft.

Per serving: Calories 193 (From Fat 120); Fat 13g (Saturated 11g); Cholesterol 23mg; Sodium 33mg; Carbohydrate 16g (Dietary Fiber 3g); Protein 2g.

Blueberry Cheesecake Ice Cream

Prep time: 20 min • **Cook time:** 5 min • **Yield:** 1½ quarts

Ingredients	Directions
1 cup raw cashews	**1** In a food processor, pulse the cashews until they're creamy, scraping the sides of the bowl as needed.
1 tablespoon lemon juice	
4 tablespoons arrowroot powder	**2** Add the lemon juice to the cashew butter and pulse to combine.
Two 13.5-ounce cans full-fat coconut milk	**3** In a medium saucepan, whisk the arrowroot powder and coconut milk until the arrowroot is dissolved. Add the cashew butter, eggs, and honey, and whisk to combine ingredients.
2 large eggs	
4 tablespoons raw honey	
1 tablespoon vanilla extract	**4** Bring the mixture to boil slowly over medium heat, stirring frequently. Remove it from the heat; let it cool for 5 minutes and then mix in the vanilla extract and refrigerate overnight.
2 cups fresh or thawed frozen blueberries	
	5 Place the mixture in an ice cream maker and process it according to the manufacturer's instructions until it reaches a soft-serve consistency.
	6 Mash the blueberries slightly and swirl them into the ice cream.
	7 Serve immediately or spoon into an airtight container and freeze until firm, about 2 hours.

Tip: You can use ½ cup of store-bought cashew butter and skip Step 1 if you prefer.

Per serving: Calories 227 (From Fat 146); Fat 16g (Saturated 11g); Cholesterol 31mg; Sodium 30mg; Carbohydrate 17g (Dietary Fiber 1g); Protein 4g.

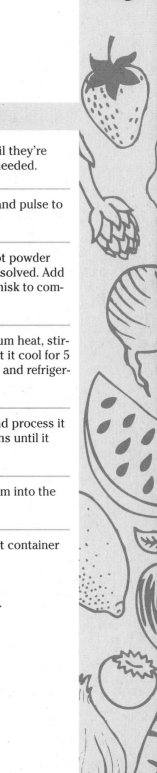

Maple-Walnut Ice Cream

Prep time: 10 min, plus overnight • **Cook time**: 5 min • **Yield**: 1 quart

Ingredients	Directions
One 13.5-ounce can full-fat coconut milk	**1** In a medium saucepan, whisk the coconut milk, egg, arrowroot powder, and salt.
1 egg	
2 tablespoons arrowroot powder	**2** Heat mixture over medium heat, stirring frequently until it starts to boil and thickens. Let the mixture cool for 5 minutes and then stir in the maple syrup and vanilla and refrigerate overnight.
Pinch of salt	
1½ teaspoons vanilla extract	
½ cup walnuts, finely chopped	**3** Place the mixture in an ice cream maker and process according to the manufacturer's instructions until it reaches a soft-serve consistency, then stir the walnuts into the ice cream.
⅓ cup maple syrup	
	4 Serve immediately or spoon into an airtight container and freeze until firm, about 2 hours.

Tip: For an extra maple flavor, drizzle top of ice cream with maple syrup before serving.

Per serving: Calories 185 (From Fat 125); Fat 14g (Saturated 8g); Cholesterol 23mg; Sodium 40mg; Carbohydrate 14g (Dietary Fiber 1g); Protein 3g.

Blueberry Vanilla Yogurt Popsicles

Prep time: 20 min, plus freezing time • **Cook time**: 5 min • **Yield**: 8 servings

Ingredients	Directions
One 13.5-ounce can full-fat coconut milk	**1** In a medium saucepan, whisk the coconut milk, arrowroot powder, and honey.
2 tablespoons arrowroot powder	**2** Heat the mixture over medium heat until it simmers and thickens, stirring constantly. Let it cool for 5 minutes and then mix in the vanilla extract and ground vanilla.
2 tablespoons raw honey	
1½ teaspoons vanilla extract	
⅛ teaspoon ground vanilla bean	**3** Divide 1 cup of the mixture evenly into 8 popsicle molds, filling each mold about ⅓ full. Freeze for about 1 hour.
1½ cups fresh or thawed frozen blueberries	**4** In a blender, combine the blueberries with the reserved coconut milk mixture and blend until smooth.
	5 Fill the popsicle molds to the top with the blueberry mixture and insert a wooden stick in each.
	6 Freeze for 4 to 6 hours, or until frozen.
	7 To remove the popsicles from the molds, dip the molds in a bowl of warm water for 30 seconds.

Tip: If you can't find ground vanilla bean, you can use another ½ teaspoon of vanilla extract instead.

Per serving: Calories 127 (From Fat 77); Fat 9g (Saturated 7g); Cholesterol 0mg; Sodium 13mg; Carbohydrate 12g (Dietary Fiber 1g); Protein 1g.

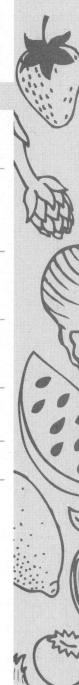

Chocolate Hazelnut Layered Ice Cream Pops

Prep time: 30 min, plus freezing time • **Cook time:** 5 min • **Yield:** 5 servings

Ingredients	Directions
One 13.5-ounce can full-fat coconut milk	**1** In a medium saucepan, whisk the coconut milk, arrowroot powder, egg, and honey.
1 egg	
2 tablespoons arrowroot powder	**2** Heat mixture slowly over medium heat until it starts to bubble and thickens, stirring frequently. Let the mixture cool for 5 minutes and then mix in the vanilla and refrigerate overnight.
2 tablespoons raw honey	
2 teaspoons vanilla extract	
⅓ cup raw or roasted hazelnuts, chopped	**3** Place the mixture in an ice cream maker and process according to the manufacturer's instructions until it reaches a soft-serve consistency. This takes about 13 minutes.
2 cups Homemade Chocolate Hazelnut Spread	
	4 Put a layer of ice cream on the bottom of 5 small (4-ounce) paper cups. Add a layer of the chopped hazelnuts and then the homemade chocolate hazelnut spread. Repeat the order until the cups are full.
	5 Place a wooden stick in the center of each cup and freeze until set, approximately 4 hours.
	6 To remove ice cream from the cups, simply tear the paper cup.

Per serving: Calories 723 (From Fat 513); Fat 57g (Saturated 19g); Cholesterol 37mg; Sodium 78mg; Carbohydrate 40g (Dietary Fiber 11g); Protein 18g.

Mint Chocolate Chip Ice Cream

Prep time: 35 min, plus overnight • **Cook time:** 5 min • **Yield:** 2 quarts

Ingredients	Directions
Two 13.5-ounce cans full-fat coconut milk	*1* Whisk the coconut milk and arrowroot powder in a medium saucepan until the arrowroot is dissolved.
4 tablespoons arrowroot powder	*2* Whisk in the honey, eggs, salt and mint, and slowly bring the mixture to a boil over medium heat, stirring frequently.
6 tablespoons raw honey	
2 eggs	
Pinch of salt	*3* When the mixture starts to bubble, remove it from heat; mix in the vanilla and let the mixture cool completely. Refrigerate the mixture overnight to infuse the mint flavor.
2 cups fresh mint leaves	
1 tablespoon vanilla extract	
1 cup Paleo-friendly dark chocolate, chopped	*4* Strain the chilled ice cream to remove the mint, pressing down firmly with a spatula to extract as much mint flavor and color as possible. Discard the mint left in the strainer.
	5 Fold in the chocolate and freeze the mixture in an ice cream maker according to the manufacturer's instructions until it reaches a soft-serve consistency.
	6 Serve immediately or spoon into an airtight container and freeze until firm, about 2 hours.

Vary It! If you want to make your own dark chocolate for this recipe, you can use the 84-percent Dark Chocolate Sweetened with Honey recipe from Chapter 7, with these modifications: Double the recipe and skip the tempering process. Line a small square dish with parchment paper, pour in the melted chocolate, and cover and freeze the pan. After the chocolate hardens, chop it into small pieces and return it to the freezer until ready to use in the ice cream. At this point, you can use it as directed in Step 5 of this recipe.

Per serving: Calories 217 (From Fat 137); Fat 15g (Saturated 11g); Cholesterol 24mg; Sodium 36mg; Carbohydrate 18g (Dietary Fiber 2g); Protein 3g.

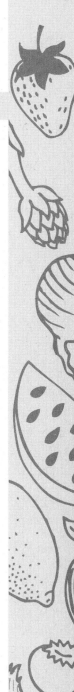

Butter Pecan Caramel Ice Cream

Prep time: 20 min, plus overnight • **Cook time:** 10 min • **Yield:** 1 quart

Ingredients	Directions
One 13.5-ounce can full-fat coconut milk	*1* Combine the coconut milk, egg, arrowroot powder, honey, and salt in a medium saucepan and slowly bring the mixture to a light boil, stirring frequently.
1 large egg	
2 tablespoons arrowroot powder	*2* Let the mixture cool for 5 minutes and then mix in the vanilla and refrigerate overnight.
3 tablespoons raw honey	
Pinch of salt	*3* Sauté the pecans in the butter until they're golden and fragrant.
1½ teaspoons vanilla extract	
½ cup pecans, coarsely chopped	*4* Place the mixture in an ice cream maker and process according to the manufacturer's instructions until it reaches a soft-serve consistency.
1 tablespoon pastured butter	
Caramel Sauce	*5* Swirl the pecans and the Caramel Sauce into the ice cream with a knife and serve immediately or spoon into an airtight container and freeze until firm, about 2 hours.

Tip: The recipe for Caramel Sauce is in Chapter 11. Make sure the caramel sauce is chilled before using; otherwise, it will melt everything and ruin your ice cream.

Per serving: Calories 246 (From Fat 158); Fat 18g (Saturated 11g); Cholesterol 27mg; Sodium 64mg; Carbohydrate 22g (Dietary Fiber 1g); Protein 2g.

Chocolate Ice Cream

Prep time: 15 min, plus overnight • **Cook time:** 5 min • **Yield:** 1 quart

Ingredients	Directions
2 ounces 100 percent Paleo-friendly dark, unsweetened chocolate	*1* Chop the dark chocolate into very small pieces.
1½ cups unsweetened shredded coconut	*2* Let the shredded coconut and water soak in a high-speed blender for 5 minutes.
3 cups hot water	*3* Blend the mixture on high for 1 minute and then strain it through a fine mesh strainer or cheesecloth into a medium saucepan (this process yields 2½ cups of coconut milk).
2 tablespoons arrowroot powder	
3 tablespoons raw cacao powder	*4* Whisk in the arrowroot powder, cacao powder, honey, and salt with the coconut milk. Bring mixture to a light boil slowly over medium heat, stirring frequently.
3 tablespoons raw honey	
Pinch of salt	*5* When the mixture starts to bubble, remove it from the heat and stir in the chocolate and vanilla until the chocolate is fully melted. Set aside to cool and then refrigerate overnight.
1 tablespoon vanilla extract	
	6 Place the mixture in and ice cream maker and process it according to the manufacturer's instructions until it reaches a soft-serve consistency.
	7 Serve immediately or spoon into an airtight container and freeze until firm, about 2 hours.

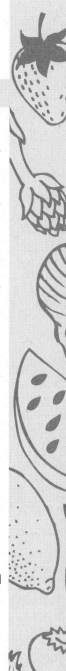

Tip: You can use 2½ cups canned full-fat coconut milk instead of making your own in Steps 2 and 3. Also, add more honey if you prefer your ice cream sweeter, or drizzle it with the Caramel Sauce from Chapter 11.

Per serving: Calories 204(From Fat 140); Fat 16g (Saturated 13g); Cholesterol 0mg; Sodium 24mg; Carbohydrate 15g (Dietary Fiber 4g); Protein 3g.

Thick and Creamy Mint Chocolate "Milkshake"

Prep time: 5 min • **Yield:** 2 servings

Ingredients	Directions
1 cup very cold water	**1** Blend all ingredients except the chocolate in a high-speed blender until everything is well combined and creamy. If you prefer a thinner milkshake, add a little bit more water until the shake reaches your desired consistency.
1 cup chopped ripe banana, (about 1 large banana) frozen	
½ cup raw cacao powder	
⅓ cup almond butter	
⅛ to ¼ teaspoon mint extract	**2** Sprinkle the top of the shake with the chocolate (if desired) and serve.
1 teaspoon vanilla extract	
Dark Paleo-friendly chopped dark chocolate (optional)	

Tip: Add some crushed ice to the blender if you like a colder shake.

Per serving: Calories 474 (From Fat 285); Fat 32g (Saturated 9g); Cholesterol 0mg; Sodium 105mg; Carbohydrate 35g (Dietary Fiber 12g); Protein 16g.

Lychee Ice Cream

Prep time: 20 min, plus overnight • **Cook time:** 10 min • **Yield:** 1½ quarts

Ingredients	Directions
1 cup fresh lychees, peeled and pitted **One 13.5-ounce can full-fat coconut milk** **1 cup heavy cream** **2 tablespoons arrowroot powder** **3 tablespoons raw honey** **1 egg, whisked** **Pinch of salt** **1½ teaspoons vanilla extract**	*1* In a medium saucepan over medium heat, heat the lychees for a couple of minutes and mash them gently with a potato masher or fork to break up the fruit.
	2 Add the coconut milk, heavy cream, arrowroot powder, honey, egg, and salt and whisk until the arrowroot is completely dissolved and everything is combined.
	3 Continue to heat the mixture, stirring constantly, until it thickens. The mixture will reach the correct thickness just as it reaches the boiling point.
	4 Remove the mixture from the stove and stir in the vanilla. Allow the mixture to cool for 1 hour and then refrigerate it overnight.
	5 Freeze mixture in an ice cream maker according to the manufacturer's instructions until it reaches a soft-serve consistency.
	6 Serve immediately or spoon into an airtight container and freeze until firm, about 2 hours.

Per serving: Calories 166 (From Fat 122); Fat 14g (Saturated 10g); Cholesterol 43mg; Sodium 34mg; Carbohydrate 11g (Dietary Fiber 0g); Protein 2g.

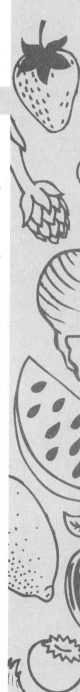

Creamy Passion Fruit Popsicles

Prep time: 15 min, plus freezing time • **Cook time:** 5 min • **Yield:** 10 servings

Ingredients	Directions
Pulp (including seeds) from 8 passion fruit, about 1⅓ cups, divided	**1** Reserve ¼ cup of passion fruit pulp and add the remaining pulp and the coconut milk to a blender.
One 13.5-ounce can full-fat coconut milk	**2** Blend for a minute or so and then strain the mixture through a fine mesh strainer into a medium saucepan.
2 tablespoons arrowroot powder	**3** Whisk in the arrowroot powder until dissolved. Mix in the coconut sugar, egg, reserved passion fruit pulp, and salt.
3 tablespoons organic coconut palm sugar	
1 egg	**4** Heat the mixture slowly over medium heat, stirring constantly, until it starts to bubble and thickens. Let it cool for 5 minutes.
Pinch of salt	
	5 Fill 10 popsicle molds with the mixture; insert wooden sticks and freeze until the popsicles are solid, about 5 hours.
	6 To release popsicles from the mold, dip the molds in a bowl of warm water for 30 seconds.

Tip: If you don't like the crunchy seeds in your popsicles, blend all of the pulp in Step 2 and strain the seeds.

Per serving: Calories 111 (From Fat 66); Fat 7g (Saturated 6g); Cholesterol 17mg; Sodium 37mg; Carbohydrate 11g (Dietary Fiber 2g); Protein 1g.

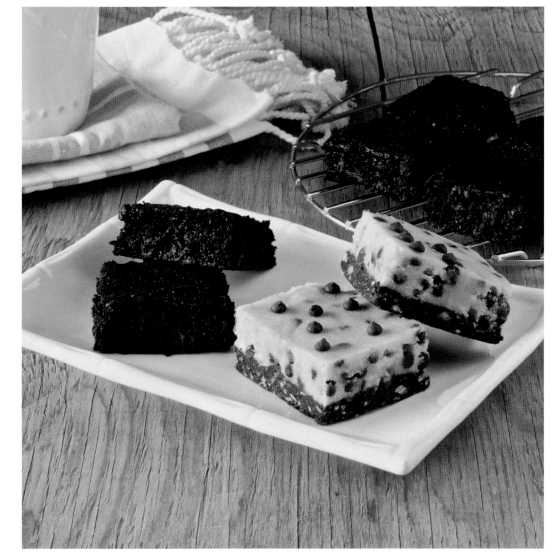

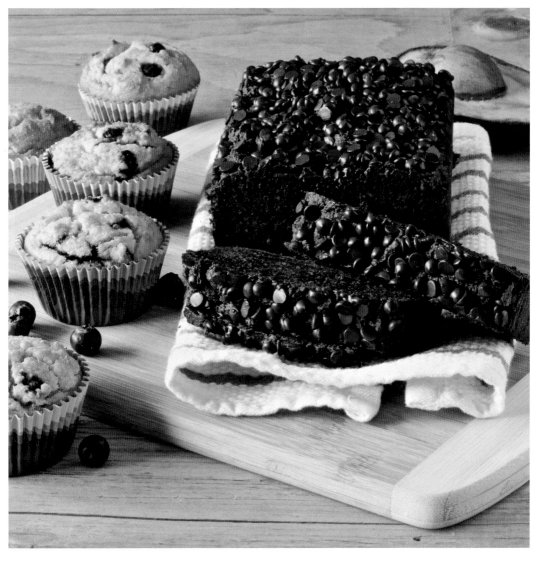

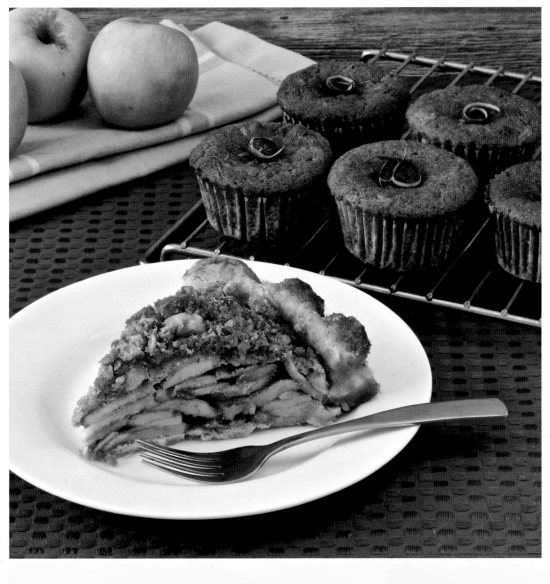

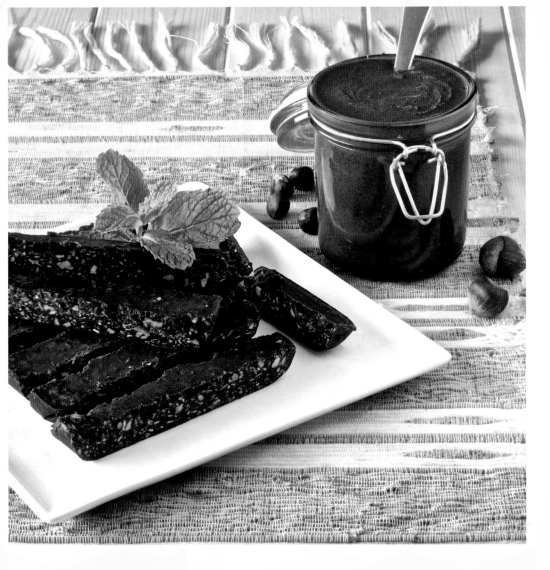

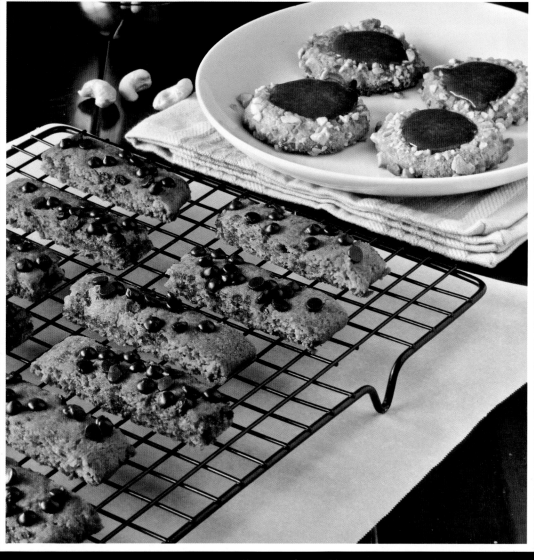

Yummy Paleo cookies.

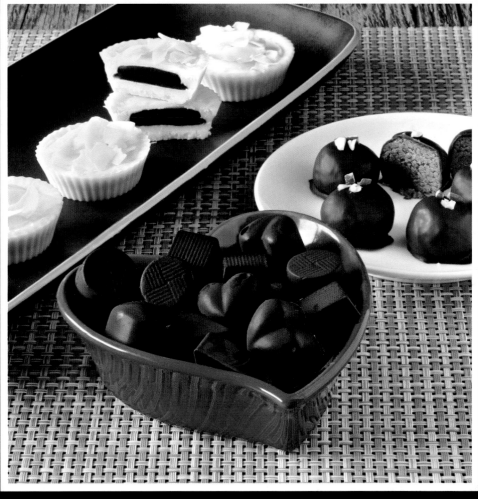

Chocolates.

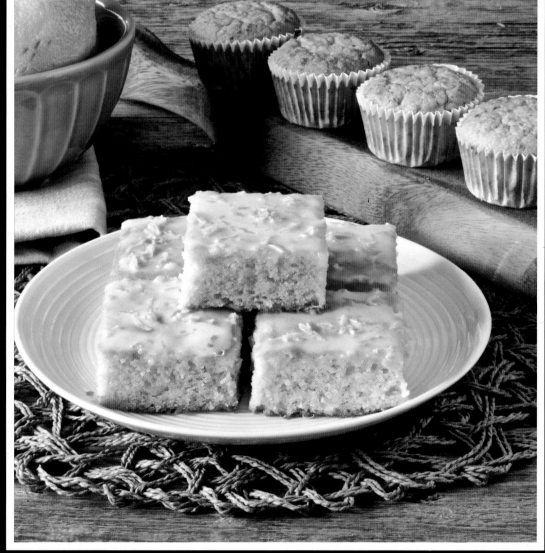

Lemon brownies and muffins.

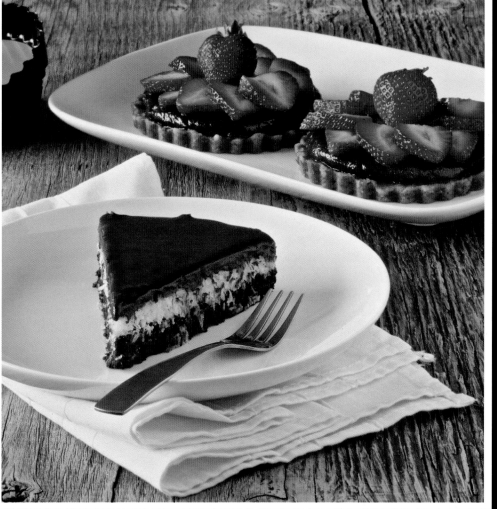

Coconut cake and strawberry tarts.

Chocolate Chip Cookie Dough Popsicles

Prep time: 15 min, plus freezing time • **Cook time:** 5 min • **Yield:** 9 servings

Ingredients	Directions
1 tablespoon arrowroot powder	**1** In a medium saucepan, whisk the almond milk and arrowroot powder until dissolved.
One 13.5-ounce can full-fat coconut milk	
1 cup almond milk	**2** Stir in the coconut milk, coconut sugar, and salt and heat the mixture over medium heat until it starts to boil. Let the mixture cool completely and then mix in the vanilla.
3 tablespoons organic coconut palm sugar	
Pinch of salt	**3** Place ½ to 1 tablespoon of chocolate chips in the bottom of each of 9 popsicle molds. Fill the molds approximately ¾ full with the milk mixture. Freeze for about 30 minutes then top them with a few additional chocolate chips.
2 teaspoons vanilla extract	
½ cup Paleo-friendly chocolate chips	
	4 Insert wooden sticks and freeze until the popsicles are solid, about 5 hours.
	5 To remove the popsicles from the molds, dip the molds in a bowl of warm water for 30 seconds.

Tip: Try using homemade almond milk in this recipe. Blend ½ cup of raw almonds and 1 cup of warm water in a blender and then strain the milk with a fine mesh strainer or cheesecloth into a saucepan. This recipe yields approximately 1 cup of almond milk.

Per serving: Calories 210 (From Fat 137); Fat 15g (Saturated 9g); Cholesterol 0mg; Sodium 28mg; Carbohydrate 16g (Dietary Fiber 2g); Protein 3g.

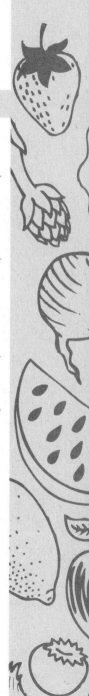

Brownie Ice Cream Cake

Prep time: 20 min, plus overnight • **Cook time:** 5 min • **Yield:** 1 quarts

Ingredients	*Directions*
One 13.5-ounce can full-fat coconut milk	**1** Combine the coconut milk, egg, arrowroot powder, honey, and salt in a medium saucepan.
1 large egg	
2 tablespoons arrowroot powder	**2** Heat the mixture until it starts to boil and becomes thicker, stirring constantly.
3 tablespoons raw honey	
1 vanilla bean	**3** Split the vanilla bean lengthwise and scrape out the seeds. Place the bean and seeds in the mixture; let it cool for a few minutes and then refrigerate it overnight.
Dash of salt	
	4 Remove the vanilla bean from the chilled mixture. Freeze the mixture in an ice cream maker according to the manufacturer's instructions until it reaches a soft-serve consistency.
	5 Serve immediately or spoon into an airtight container and freeze until firm, about 2 hours.

Brownie

Prep time: 20 min, plus freezing time • **Yield:** 8 servings

Ingredients	Directions
5 large Medjool dates, pitted	**1** Process the dates into a creamy paste in a food processor. Pulse in the almond flour, cacao powder, vanilla, and coconut oil. Pulse in the chopped pecans.
½ cup blanched almond flour	
4 tablespoons raw cacao powder	
½ teaspoon vanilla extract	**2** Spread the mixture evenly onto the bottom of two 4-x-1¾-inch mini springform pans.
½ tablespoon coconut oil, melted	
⅓ cup pecans, chopped plus additional for garnish	**3** Spread the Vanilla Ice Cream over the brownie and freeze for about 2 hours.
Vanilla Ice Cream (see the earlier recipe)	**4** Remove the cakes from the springform pans, top them with the Chocolate Fudge Topping and chopped pecans, and serve.
Chocolate Fudge Topping	

Tip: Look for the Vanilla Ice Cream recipe earlier in this chapter and the Chocolate Fudge Topping recipe in Chapter 11.

Per serving: Calories 304 (From Fat 183); Fat 20g (Saturated 12g); Cholesterol 23mg; Sodium 48mg; Carbohydrate 30g (Dietary Fiber 4g); Protein 5g.

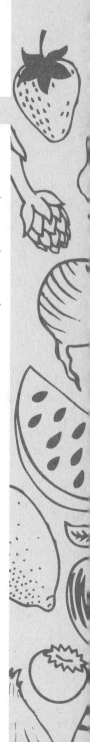

Coconut Popsicles

Prep time: 15 min, plus overnight • **Cook time:** 5 min • **Yield:** 8 servings

Ingredients	Directions
2 tablespoons water	*1* Add the water to a large bowl and sprinkle the gelatin on top.
½ teaspoon unflavored gelatin (preferably made from pastured cows)	
One 13.5-ounce can full-fat coconut milk	*2* Gently bring the coconut milk to a boil over medium heat. Pour the boiling milk into the bowl with the gelatin and whisk until the gelatin dissolves.
2 to 3 tablespoons raw honey	*3* Whisk in the honey, vanilla, and salt.
1 teaspoon vanilla extract	
Pinch of salt	*4* Distribute the coconut flakes evenly into 8 popsicle molds and then fill each to the top with the coconut milk mixture. Insert wooden sticks and freeze overnight.
½ cup unsweetened dried coconut flakes	
	5 To remove the popsicles from the molds, dip the molds in a bowl of warm water for 30 seconds.

Tip: If you can find mature coconuts in your grocery store, consider substituting chopped fresh coconut meat in place of the flakes in Step 4.

Per serving: Calories 120 (From Fat 91); Fat 10g (Saturated 9g); Cholesterol 0mg; Sodium 31mg; Carbohydrate 7g (Dietary Fiber 1g); Protein 1g.

Toasted Coconut Caramel Ice Cream

Prep time: 15 min, plus overnight • **Cook time:** 5 min • **Yield:** 1 quart

Ingredients	Directions
½ cup unsweetened shredded coconut	*1* Preheat the oven to 300 degrees. Toast the shredded coconut for about 2 minutes, being careful not to burn it.
1 13.5-ounce can full-fat coconut milk	
2 tablespoons arrowroot powder	*2* In a medium saucepan, whisk the coconut milk and arrowroot powder and then mix in the egg, honey, and salt.
1 egg	
2 tablespoons raw honey	*3* Heat the mixture slowly over medium heat, stirring frequently until it starts to boil and thickens.
Pinch of salt	
1 teaspoon vanilla extract	*4* Remove the mixture from the stove and mix in the toasted coconut and the vanilla. Refrigerate the mixture overnight.
Homemade Caramel Sauce, chilled	
	5 Freeze mixture in an ice cream maker according to the manufacturer's instructions until it reaches a soft-serve consistency. Swirl in the Homemade Caramel Sauce.
	6 Serve immediately or spoon into an airtight container and freeze until firm, about 2 hours.

Per serving: Calories 221 (From Fat 139); Fat 15g (Saturated 13g); Cholesterol 23mg; Sodium 66mg; Carbohydrate 20g (Dietary Fiber 1g); Protein 2g.

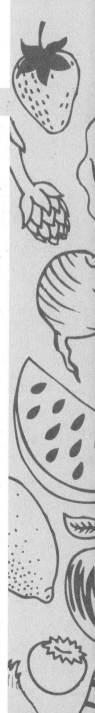

Honey-Roasted Macadamia Nut Ice Cream

Prep time: 25 min, plus overnight • **Cook time:** 20 min • **Yield:** 1 quart

Ingredients	Directions
Honey Roasted Macadamia Nuts (see the following recipe)	**1** Blend the raw macadamia nuts and the water in a blender for a couple of minutes. Strain the mixture through a fine mesh strainer or cheesecloth into a saucepan to yield 1 cup of macadamia nut milk.
½ cup raw macadamia nuts	
1 cup warm water	
2 tablespoons arrowroot powder	**2** Whisk the arrowroot powder into the nut milk until dissolved.
1½ cups full-fat coconut milk	**3** Mix in the coconut milk, salt, honey, and egg and heat the mixture slowly over medium heat, stirring constantly until it starts to bubble and thickens.
Pinch of salt	
3 tablespoons raw honey	
1 egg	**4** Remove the mixture from the heat; let it cool for 5 minutes and then mix in the vanilla and refrigerate overnight.
1½ teaspoons vanilla extract	
	5 Freeze it in an ice cream maker according to the manufacturer's instructions until it reaches a soft-serve consistency and then stir the Honey Roasted Macadamia Nuts into the ice cream.
	6 Serve immediately or spoon into an airtight container and freeze until firm, about 2 hours.

Honey Roasted Macadamia Nuts

½ tablespoon raw honey

1 teaspoon macadamia nut oil

Pinch of salt

½ cup raw macadamia nuts, halved or chopped

1 Preheat the oven to 350 degrees. In a bowl, whisk the honey, macadamia nut oil, and salt.

2 Add the macadamia nuts and mix well until all nuts are coated.

3 Line a baking sheet with parchment paper and spread the coated nuts across the pan.

4 Bake for 15 minutes or until golden brown, being careful not to burn.

Vary It! You can use coconut oil in place of the macadamia nut oil for the roasted nuts.

Per serving *Calories 251 (From Fat 197); Fat 22g (Saturated 9g); Cholesterol 23mg; Sodium 56mg; Carbohydrate 14g (Dietary Fiber 2g); Protein 3g.*

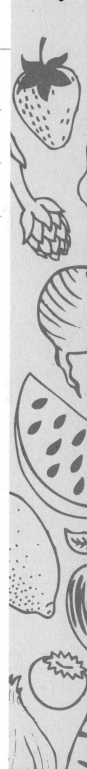

Chapter 10

Muffins and Cupcakes

One of the greatest pleasures of life is enjoying the foods you love, including sweet cupcakes and yummy muffins. No one wants to go through life following strict dietary guidelines, feeling guilty for not following every rule 100 percent of the time.

Okay, so cavemen probably weren't baking muffins or cupcakes, but that doesn't mean you have to avoid those goodies altogether. Redefining the way you make these foods — removing the bad stuff and replacing it with nutrient-rich ingredients — keeps you on a healthy track while letting you have a sweet treat now and then.

Baking Paleo muffins and cupcakes is super easy and delicious. You'll be surprised to discover how good a blueberry muffin can taste when made with almond or coconut flour and sweetened with a little raw honey. Luckily, you don't need any special equipment or a lot of time to make these recipes. A mixing bowl, a rubber spatula, a muffin pan, and about 15 minutes of your day are all that they require. So take a tour through this chapter and bake up the sweet treats that sound yummiest to you.

Coconut Cupcakes

Prep time: 20 min, plus overnight • **Cook time:** 20 min • **Yield:** 6 servings

Ingredients	Directions
Coconut Whipped Cream Frosting (see the following recipe) 1 cup blanched almond flour ¼ teaspoon baking soda 3 tablespoons raw cacao powder ¼ cup unsweetened shredded coconut 2 tablespoons coconut butter 1 egg 2 tablespoons coconut oil, melted ½ cup full-fat coconut milk 2 tablespoons raw honey 1 teaspoon vanilla extract Toasted shredded coconut for garnish (optional)	**1** Preheat the oven to 350 degrees and line a muffin tin with baking cups. In a large bowl, mix the almond flour, baking soda, cacao powder, and untoasted shredded coconut. **2** In a separate bowl, whisk the coconut butter, egg, coconut oil, coconut milk, honey, and vanilla. **3** Using a rubber spatula, gently mix the dry ingredients and wet ingredients. **4** Spoon the batter into the prepared muffin tin, filling each cup to the top. **5** Bake until a toothpick inserted into the center comes out clean, about 20 minutes. Cool on a wire rack. **6** Top each muffin with the Coconut Whipped Cream Frosting and sprinkle with the toasted shredded coconut (if desired).

Coconut Whipped Cream Frosting

One 13.5-ounce can full-fat
coconut milk

1 teaspoon vanilla extract

1 Place the can of full-fat coconut milk in the fridge overnight.

2 Scoop out the solid coconut cream that forms on the top of the can and place it in a bowl. Be careful not to mix the solid coconut with the water in the bottom of the can. Discard the water.

3 Add the vanilla to the cream and whip the mixture with an electric handheld or stand mixer until fluffy.

Tip: Add a couple teaspoons of raw honey to the Coconut Whipped Cream Frosting in Step 5 for a sweeter frosting.

Per serving: Calories 407 (From Fat 322); Fat 36g (Saturated 23g); Cholesterol 31mg; Sodium 96mg; Carbohydrate 17g (Dietary Fiber 4g); Protein 7g.

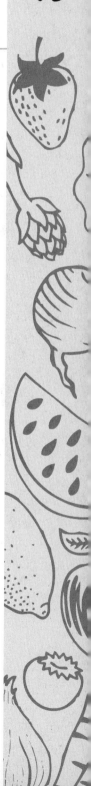

Red Velvet Cupcakes with Coconut Whipped Cream Frosting

Prep time: 20 min, plus overnight • **Cook time:** 30–35 min • **Yield:** 6 servings

Ingredients	Directions
Coconut Whipped Cream Frosting (see the following recipe)	*1* Preheat the oven to 350 degrees and line a muffin tin with 6 baking cups. Mix the almond flour, baking soda, and raw cacao powder in a bowl.
1¼ cups blanched almond flour	
½ teaspoon baking soda	*2* In a separate bowl, whisk the coconut oil, coconut milk, vanilla, vinegar, honey, egg, and beets.
2 tablespoons raw cacao powder	
¼ cup coconut oil, melted	*3* Using a rubber spatula, gently mix the wet ingredients and dry ingredients. Fold in the chocolate chips.
7 tablespoons full-fat coconut milk	
1 teaspoon vanilla extract	*4* Spoon the batter into the prepared muffin tin, filling each cup to the top.
1 teaspoon apple cider vinegar	
2 tablespoons raw honey	*5* Bake until a toothpick inserted into the center comes out clean, about 30 to 35 minutes.
1 egg	
¼ cup finely grated peeled beets	*6* Set the pan on a wire rack to cool and then top the cupcakes with the Coconut Whipped Cream Frosting and a fresh cherry.
¼ cup Paleo-friendly chocolate chips	
6 fresh cherries, pitted	

Coconut Whipped Cream Frosting

One 13.5-ounce can full-fat coconut milk

1 teaspoon vanilla extract

1 Place the can of full-fat coconut milk in the fridge overnight.

2 Scoop the coconut cream that forms on top of the can into a bowl, being careful not to mix with the water in the bottom of the can. Discard the water.

3 Add the vanilla and use an electric handheld or stand mixer to whip the coconut cream until fluffy.

Tip: When grating the beet, be sure to use the fine holes in the greater.

Per serving: Calories 467 (From Fat 356); Fat 40g (Saturated 24g); Cholesterol 31mg; Sodium 150mg; Carbohydrate 23g (Dietary Fiber 4g); Protein 9g.

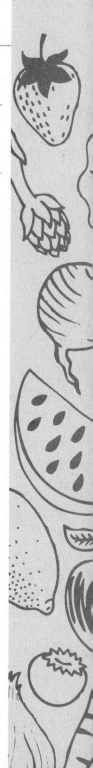

Strawberry-Stuffed Chocolate Cupcakes

Prep time: 20 min • **Cook time:** 22 min • **Yield:** 6 servings

Ingredients	Directions
Chocolate Frosting (see the following recipe)	*1* Preheat the oven to 350 degrees and line a muffin tin with baking cups. Melt the chocolate chips in a bowl over simmering water (double boiler) and let it cool for 5 minutes.
¼ cup Paleo-friendly chocolate chips	
1 egg	*2* Whisk the egg, coconut oil, coconut milk, and honey into the melted chocolate until smooth.
2 tablespoons coconut oil, melted	
⅓ cup full-fat coconut milk	*3* In a large bowl, mix the almond flour, cacao powder, and baking soda.
1 to 2 tablespoon raw honey	
1¾ cup blanched almond flour	*4* Using a rubber spatula, gently mix the wet ingredients and dry ingredients to form a batter.
1 tablespoon raw cacao powder	
2 teaspoons baking soda	*5* Spoon the batter into the prepared muffin tin, filling each cup to the top.
6 fresh strawberries	
	6 Cut the tops off 6 strawberries and insert one in each cupcake, pointy side down.
	7 Bake until a toothpick inserted into the edges of the muffin comes out clean, about 22 minutes.
	8 Allow the cupcakes to cool on a wire rack before frosting. Top each cupcake with the Chocolate Frosting. Store any uneaten cupcakes in the fridge.

Chocolate Frosting

¾ **cup Paleo-friendly chocolate chips**

6 tablespoons full-fat coconut milk

1 Melt the chocolate chips in a bowl over simmering water (double boiler).

2 Mix the coconut milk with the melted chocolate until smooth.

Per serving: Calories 520 (From Fat 360); Fat 40g (Saturated 18g); Cholesterol 31mg; Sodium 451mg; Carbohydrate 37g (Dietary Fiber 7g); Protein 11g.

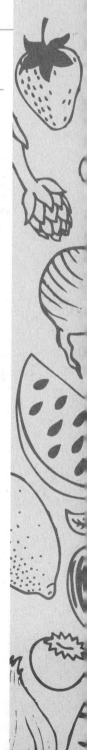

Vanilla Cupcakes with Chocolate-Banana Frosting

Prep time: 25 min • **Cook time:** 20 min • **Yield:** 6 servings

Ingredients	Directions
Chocolate Banana Frosting (see the following recipe)	*1* Preheat the oven to 350 degrees and line a muffin tin with 6 baking cups. Mix the almond flour, baking soda, and salt in a bowl.
1½ cups blanched almond flour	
1¼ teaspoons baking soda	*2* In a separate bowl, whisk the coconut milk, coconut oil, vanilla, honey, and eggs.
½ teaspoon salt	
½ cup full-fat coconut milk	*3* Using a rubber spatula, gently mix the wet ingredients and dry ingredients. Don't overmix.
2 tablespoons coconut oil, melted	
2 teaspoons vanilla extract	*4* Spoon the batter into the prepared muffin tin, filling each to the top. Bake until a toothpick inserted into the center comes out clean, about 20 minutes. Set the pan on a wire rack to cool.
3 tablespoons raw honey	
2 room temperature eggs	*5* Cut a small hole in the center of each muffin. Using a piping bag, squeeze about 2 teaspoons of the Chocolate Banana Frosting into the center of each muffin and then frost the tops of the muffins. Store muffins and frosting in an airtight container in the fridge for 1 to 2 weeks.

Chocolate Banana Frosting

⅓ **cup cacao butter**

2½ **cups chopped bananas**

1½ **cups raw cacao powder**

5 **tablespoons raw honey**

2 **teaspoons vanilla extract**

1 Melt the cacao butter in a bowl over simmering water (double boiler).

2 In a food processor, pulse the melted cacao butter with the remaining ingredients until creamy and smooth.

Tip: If you don't have a piping bag, you can make one out of a plastic baggie. Put the frosting in the baggie, working it into one corner. Snip off that corner and boom — instant piping bag. Bonus: You can just throw it away when you're done.

Tip: Apple bananas enhance the flavor of this frosting, so consider using them if you can find them at your local stores or online.

Per serving: *Calories 545 (From Fat 324); Fat 36g (Saturated 17g); Cholesterol 62mg; Sodium 499mg; Carbohydrate 52g (Dietary Fiber 6g); Protein 10g.*

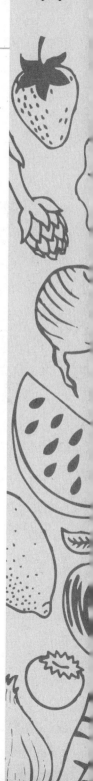

Banana Chocolate Chip Muffins with Cinnamon Streusel

Prep time: 20 min • **Cook time:** 15 min • **Yield:** 10 servings

Ingredients	Directions
Cinnamon Streusel (see the following recipe)	**1** Preheat the oven to 350 degrees and line a muffin tin with 10 baking cups. Chop the pecans in a food processor until they form a coarse meal.
½ cup raw pecans	
1½ cups blanched almond flour	**2** In a large bowl, mix the chopped pecans, almond flour, cinnamon, baking soda, and salt.
½ teaspoon ground cinnamon	
1½ teaspoons baking soda	**3** Pulse the bananas, egg, honey, coconut oil, and coconut cream in a food processor until creamy.
½ teaspoon salt	
1½ cups chopped bananas	**4** Using a rubber spatula, gently mix the banana mixture with the dry ingredients to form a batter; fold in the chocolate chips, reserving a few for garnish. Don't overmix.
1 egg	
1 tablespoon raw honey	
3 tablespoons coconut oil, melted	**5** Spoon the batter into the prepared muffin tin, filling each cup to the top.
3 tablespoons coconut cream	
⅓ cup Paleo-friendly chocolate chips, plus a few extra	**6** Top each muffin with the Cinnamon Streusel and a few of the reserved chocolate chips and bake until a toothpick inserted into the center comes out clean, approximately 15 minutes.
	7 Set the muffin pan on a wire rack to cool.

Cinnamon Streusel

2 tablespoons blanched almond flour

⅛ teaspoon ground cinnamon

1¼ teaspoons coconut oil, melted

1   Mix all ingredients until crumbly.

Tip: Coconut cream is the thick cream that forms on the top of a can of full-fat coconut milk when you leave it in the fridge overnight, discarding the water.

Tip: Apple bananas enhance the flavor of these muffins, so consider using them if you can find them at your local stores or online. Apple bananas are smaller than the more common varieties and have a distinct sweet yet tangy flavor. As they ripen, they become sweeter and develop a unique tropical flavor resembling a blend of pineapple and strawberries. They grow year round in tropical regions and are readily available in Hawaii, Honduras, Malaysia, and Mexico.

Per serving: Calories 279 (From Fat 197); Fat 22g (Saturated 8g); Cholesterol 19mg; Sodium 319mg; Carbohydrate 19g (Dietary Fiber 4g); Protein 6g.

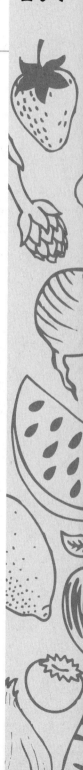

Flourless Chocolate Hazelnut Muffins

Prep time: 20 min • **Cook time:** 12–15 min • **Yield:** 9 servings

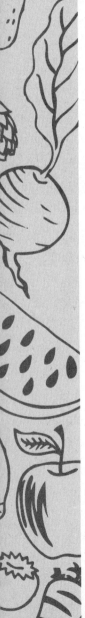

Ingredients	Directions
2½ cups raw hazelnuts, blanched **½ cup raw cacao powder** **½ teaspoon baking soda** **¼ cup Paleo-friendly dark chocolate chips** **½ cup chopped bananas** **2 room temperature eggs** **3 tablespoons raw honey** **1 teaspoon apple cider vinegar** **½ teaspoon vanilla extract** **Whole hazelnuts and extra chocolate chips, if desired**	**1** Preheat the oven to 350 degrees and line a muffin tin with 9 baking cups. Set aside 6 whole hazelnuts. Process the remaining hazelnuts in a food processor or high-speed blender until creamy and smooth and has a liquid-like consistency.
	2 Place this hazelnut butter in a large bowl; mix in the cacao powder and baking soda with a rubber spatula until fully combined.
	3 Process the bananas, eggs, honey, vinegar, and vanilla in a food processor until smooth. Add this mixture to the hazelnut mixture and mix it with a rubber spatula until fully combined into a thick batter.
	4 Spoon the batter into the prepared muffin tin, filling each cup to the top.
	5 Smooth the top of each muffin with the back of a spoon, place a reserved hazelnut in the center of each muffin, and sprinkle the tops with the reserved chocolate chips (if desired).
	6 Bake until a toothpick inserted into the center comes out clean, about 12 to 15 minutes.
	7 Allow the muffins to cool on a wire rack.

Tip: Apple bananas enhance the flavor of these muffins, so consider using them if you can find them at your local stores or online.

Tip: Instead of grinding up whole hazelnuts in Step 1, you can skip that task and substitute 1 cup of store-bought hazelnut butter in Step 2.

Per serving: Calories 347 (From Fat 255); Fat 28g (Saturated 5g); Cholesterol 41mg; Sodium 88mg; Carbohydrate 21g (Dietary Fiber 6g); Protein 9g.

Lemon Chia Seed Muffins

Prep time: 15 min • **Cook time:** 30–35 min • **Yield:** 6 servings

Ingredients	Directions
⅓ cup coconut flour	**1** Preheat the oven to 350 degrees and line a muffin tin with 6 baking cups. Mix the coconut flour, tapioca flour, baking soda, chia seeds, and salt in a bowl.
¼ cup tapioca flour	
⅛ teaspoon baking soda	
1 tablespoon chia seeds	**2** In a separate bowl, whisk the remaining ingredients.
¼ teaspoon salt	
2 tablespoons coconut oil, melted	**3** Using a rubber spatula, mix the wet ingredients and dry ingredients to form a batter.
½ cup full-fat canned coconut milk	**4** Pour the batter into the prepared muffin tin, filling each cup to the top.
3 eggs	
3 tablespoons maple syrup	**5** Bake until a toothpick inserted into the center comes out clean, about 20 to 30 minutes.
1 tablespoon lemon juice	
2 teaspoons lemon zest	**6** Set the pan over a wire rack to cool.
1 teaspoon vanilla extract	

Per serving: Calories 191 (From Fat 105); Fat 12g (Saturated 9g); Cholesterol 93mg; Sodium 179mg; Carbohydrate 17g (Dietary Fiber 3g); Protein 5g.

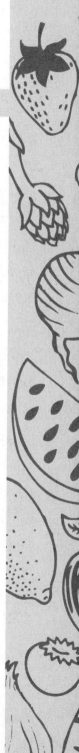

Flourless Chocolate Chip Muffins

Prep time: 10 min • **Cook time:** 25 min • **Yield:** 8 servings

Ingredients	Directions
3 tablespoons raw honey	**1** Preheat the oven to 350 degrees and line a muffin tin with 8 baking cups. In a large bowl, whisk the honey, eggs, vanilla, vinegar, and baking soda.
2 eggs	
½ teaspoon vanilla extract	
1 teaspoon apple cider vinegar	**2** Mix in the almond butter using a rubber spatula and then gently fold in the chocolate chips.
½ teaspoon baking soda	
1 cup almond butter	**3** Spoon the batter into the prepared muffin tin, filling each cup to the top.
¼ cup Paleo-friendly chocolate chips	
	4 Bake until a toothpick inserted into the center comes out clean, about 25 minutes.
	5 Allow the muffins to cool on a wire rack before serving.

Tip: Consider making the almond butter at home. Add 2¼ cups of almonds to your food processor and process until creamy and smooth, scraping the sides of the bowl as needed. When using store bought almond butter, be sure to stir the content in the jar first.

Per serving: Calories 279 (From Fat 193); Fat 21g (Saturated 4g); Cholesterol 47mg; Sodium 169mg; Carbohydrate 17g (Dietary Fiber 4g); Protein 9g.

Banana Crumb Muffins

Prep time: 15 min • **Cook time:** 17 min • **Yield:** 8 servings

Ingredients	Directions
Crumb Topping (see the following recipe)	**1** Preheat the oven to 350 degrees and line a muffin tin with 8 baking cups. Mix the almond flour, baking soda, and salt in a bowl.
1½ cups blanched almond flour	
1 teaspoon baking soda	
½ teaspoon salt	**2** In a separate bowl, mash the bananas with a fork and mix in the honey, egg, and butter.
1½ cups chopped bananas	
1 tablespoon raw honey	**3** Using a rubber spatula, gently mix the wet ingredients and dry ingredients. Don't overmix. Fold in the pecans.
1 egg	
5 tablespoons pastured butter, melted	**4** Spoon the batter into the prepared muffin tin, filling each cup to the top.
⅓ cup raw pecans, chopped	
	5 Sprinkle the top of each muffin with the Crumb Topping and bake until a toothpick inserted into the center comes out clean, about 17 minutes.

Crumb Topping

2 tablespoons blanched almond flour	**1** Using your hands, mix all the ingredients until the mixture resembles coarse cornmeal.
1 tablespoon cold, pastured butter	
⅛ teaspoon ground cinnamon	

Tip: Apple bananas enhance the flavor of these muffins, so consider using them if you can find them at your local stores or online.

Per serving: Calories 269 (From Fat 212); Fat 24g (Saturated 7g); Cholesterol 46mg; Sodium 321mg; Carbohydrate 17g (Dietary Fiber 8g); Protein 7g.

Blueberry Muffins

Prep time: 15 min • **Cook time:** 30-3520–25 min • **Yield:** 6 servings

Ingredients	Directions
1 cup blanched almond flour	*1* Preheat the oven to 350 degrees and line a muffin tin with 6 baking cups.
⅛ teaspoon baking soda	
Pinch of slat	*2* Mix the almond flour, baking soda, and salt in a bowl.
2 tablespoons raw honey	
½ cup full-fat coconut milk	*3* In a separate bowl, whisk the honey, coconut milk, coconut oil, egg, and vanilla.
2 tablespoons coconut oil, melted	
1 egg	*4* Using a rubber spatula, mix the wet ingredients and dry ingredients. Don't overmix.
1 teaspoon vanilla extract	
¼ cup fresh blueberries	*5* Gently fold the blueberries into the batter.
	6 Spoon the batter into the prepared muffin tin, filling each cup to the top.
	7 Bake until a toothpick inserted into the center comes out clean, about 20-25 minutes.
	8 Set the pan on a wire rack to cool. Wait until the muffins are completely cool before removing them from the paper liners.

Note: You must use fresh blueberries in this recipe; frozen berries won't work.

Per serving: Calories 192 (From Fat 137); Fat 15g (Saturated 8g); Cholesterol 93mg; Sodium 71mg; Carbohydrate 10g (Dietary Fiber 1g); Protein 6g.

Apple Cinnamon Muffins

Prep time: 5 min • **Cook time:** 20 min • **Yield:** 5 servings

Ingredients	Directions
1½ cups blanched almond flour ½ teaspoon baking soda 1 teaspoon ground cinnamon Pinch of salt ½ cup unsweetened applesauce 1 teaspoon apple cider vinegar 1 room temperature egg 1 teaspoon vanilla extract 1 to 2 tablespoons raw honey	**1** Preheat the oven to 350 degrees and line a muffin tin with baking cups. Mix the almond flour, baking soda, cinnamon, and salt in a bowl. **2** In a separate bowl, whisk the applesauce, vinegar, egg, vanilla, and honey. **3** Spoon the batter into the prepared muffin tin, filling each cup to the top. **4** Bake until a toothpick inserted into the center comes out clean, approximately 20 minutes. **5** Allow the muffins to cool on a wire rack before serving.

Per serving: Calories 233 (From Fat 160); Fat 18g (Saturated 2g); Cholesterol 37mg; Sodium 181mg; Carbohydrate 14g (Dietary Fiber 4g); Protein 9g.

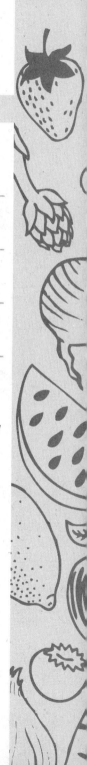

Nut-free Blueberry Muffins

Prep time: 15 min • **Cook time:** 30–35 min • **Yield:** 6 servings

Ingredients	Directions
⅓ cup plus 2 tablespoons coconut flour (about 59 grams)	**1** Preheat the oven to 350 degrees and line a muffin tin with 6 baking cups. Mix the coconut flour and baking soda in a bowl.
⅛ teaspoon baking soda	
2 tablespoons raw honey	**2** In a separate bowl, whisk the honey, coconut milk, coconut oil, eggs, and vanilla.
½ cup full-fat coconut milk	
2 tablespoons coconut oil, melted	**3** Using a rubber spatula, mix the wet ingredients and dry ingredients. Gently fold the blueberries into the batter.
3 eggs	
½ teaspoon vanilla extract	**4** Spoon the batter into the prepared muffin tin, filling each cup to the top.
¼ cup fresh blueberries	
	5 Bake until a toothpick inserted into the center comes out clean, about 30 to 35 minutes.
	6 Set the pan on a wire rack to cool. Wait until the muffins are completely cool before serving.

Note: You must use fresh blueberries in this recipe; frozen berries won't work.

Per serving: Calories 192 (From Fat 137); Fat 15g (Saturated 8g); Cholesterol 93mg; Sodium 71mg; Carbohydrate 10g (Dietary Fiber 1g); Protein 6g.

Chocolate Hazelnut Swirl Banana Muffins

Prep time: 20 min • **Cook time:** 15–17 min • **Yield:** 6 servings

Ingredients	Directions
2 cups blanched almond flour	**1** Preheat the oven to 325 degrees and line a muffin tin with 6 baking cups. Mix the almond flour, baking soda, and salt in a bowl.
2 teaspoons baking soda	
½ teaspoon salt	
1½ cups chopped bananas	**2** In a separate bowl, mash the bananas with a fork and then mix in the honey, egg, coconut oil, and vanilla.
1 to 2 tablespoons raw honey	
1 large egg	**3** Using a rubber spatula, gently mix the wet ingredients and dry ingredients. Fold in the chopped pecans.
¼ cup coconut oil, melted	
2 teaspoons vanilla extract	**4** Spoon the batter into the prepared muffin tin, filling each cup ¾ full.
½ cup pecans, chopped	
¼ cup Homemade Chocolate Hazelnut Spread	**5** Add a teaspoon of Homemade Chocolate Hazelnut Spread on top of each muffin and swirl the spread around with a toothpick or knife.
	6 Bake until a toothpick inserted into the center comes out clean, about 15 to 17 minutes.
	7 Cool completely on a wire rack before serving.

Tip: You can find the Homemade Chocolate Hazelnut Spread recipe in Chapter 11.

Tip: Apple bananas enhance the flavor of these muffins, so consider using them if you can find them at your local stores or online.

Per serving: Calories 475 (From Fat 343); Fat 39g (Saturated 11g); Cholesterol 31mg; Sodium 644mg; Carbohydrate 28g (Dietary Fiber 7g); Protein 12g.

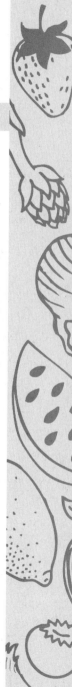

Chocolate Chip Scones

Prep time: 20 min • **Cook time:** 10–15 min • **Yield:** 10 servings

Ingredients	Directions
2 cups blanched almond flour	**1** Preheat the oven to 350 degrees. In a large bowl, mix the almond flour, arrowroot powder, coconut sugar, and salt.
¼ cup arrowroot powder	
⅓ cup organic coconut palm sugar	
½ teaspoon salt	**2** Using a fork, cut the butter into the flour mixture until it resembles coarse meal. Stir in the chocolate chips.
5 tablespoons cold, pastured butter, chopped into small pieces	**3** In a separate bowl, whisk the yogurt and egg.
½ cup Paleo-friendly chocolate chips	**4** Using a fork, stir the wet ingredients until just combined. Don't overwork; the dough should be crumbly.
1 teaspoon baking soda	**5** Transfer the dough to a baking sheet lined with parchment paper and form it into a 6-inch circle.
½ cup plain Greek yogurt	
1 egg	**6** Using a pastry cutter or knife, cut the dough into 10 wedges. Gently separate each piece on the baking sheet 2-inches apart.
	7 Bake until golden, about 10 to 15 minutes, rotating the sheet halfway through. Set the baking sheet on a wire rack and allow the scones to cool.

Per serving: Calories 294 (From Fat 195); Fat 22g (Saturated 7g); Cholesterol 35mg; Sodium 266mg; Carbohydrate 22g (Dietary Fiber 3g); Protein 8g.

Coconut Flour Banana Muffins

Prep time: 15 min • **Cook time:** 12–15 min • **Yield:** 6 servings

Ingredients	Directions
3 tablespoons coconut oil, melted	**1** Preheat the oven to 375 degrees and line a muffin tin with 6 baking cups. Mix the coconut oil, eggs, honey, bananas, shredded coconut, and vanilla in a bowl.
3 eggs	
1 tablespoon raw honey	**2** In a separate bowl, mix the coconut flour, salt, and baking soda.
1½ cups chopped ripe bananas	
¼ cup unsweetened shredded coconut	**3** Using a spatula, slowly mix the dry ingredients into the wet ingredients until thoroughly combined.
½ teaspoon vanilla extract	
¼ cup coconut flour	**4** Fold in the macadamia nuts and chocolate chips (if desired).
½ teaspoon salt	
¼ teaspoon baking soda	**5** Bake until a toothpick inserted into the center comes out clean, about 12 to 15 minutes.
¼ cup macadamia nuts, chopped (optional)	
¼ cup chocolate chips (optional)	

Tip: Apple bananas enhance the flavor of these muffins, so consider using them if you can find them at your local stores or online.

Per serving: *Calories 203 (From Fat 110); Fat 13g (Saturated 10g); Cholesterol 93mg; Sodium 294mg; Carbohydrate 20g (Dietary Fiber 4g); Protein 5g.*

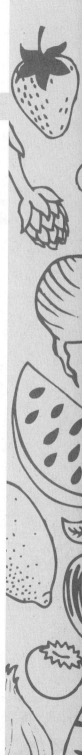

Dark Chocolate Cherry Muffins

Prep time: 15 min • **Cook time:** 20–25 min • **Yield:** 7 servings

Ingredients	Directions
¼ cup fresh sweet cherries, chopped	**1** Preheat the oven to 350 degrees and line a muffin tin with 7 baking cups. Mix the coconut flour, arrowroot powder, baking soda, and salt.
⅓ cup plus 2 tablespoons coconut flour	
1 tablespoon arrowroot powder	**2** In a separate bowl, whisk the eggs well and then whisk in the coconut milk, coconut oil, honey, and vanilla.
¼ teaspoon baking soda	
¼ teaspoon salt	**3** Using a rubber spatula, mix the wet ingredients and dry ingredients to form a thick batter. Fold in the cherries, dark chocolate, and sliced almonds (if desired).
3 eggs	
½ cup full-fat coconut milk	**4** Spoon the batter into the prepared muffin tin, filling each cup to the top.
2 tablespoons coconut oil, melted	
2 tablespoons raw honey	**5** Bake until a toothpick inserted into the center comes out clean, about 20 to 25 minutes.
¼ teaspoon ground vanilla powder	
¼ cup 70-percent dark chocolate, chopped	**6** Set the pan on a wire rack to cool.
2 tablespoons sliced almonds (optional)	

Per serving: Calories 187 (From Fat 114); Fat 13g (Saturated 9g); Cholesterol 80mg; Sodium 226mg; Carbohydrate 16g (Dietary Fiber 4g); Protein 5g.

Zucchini Muffins

Prep time: 15 min • **Cook time:** 20 min • **Yield:** 5 servings

Ingredients	*Directions*
½ cup finely grated zucchini (about 50 grams) 1 egg 3 tablespoons raw honey 1½ tablespoons fresh orange juice 2 tablespoons coconut oil, melted ¼ teaspoon vanilla extract 1 cup blanched almond flour ½ teaspoon ground cinnamon ½ teaspoon baking soda ⅛ teaspoon salt	**1** Preheat the oven to 350 degrees and line a muffin tin with 5 baking cups. Whisk the zucchini, egg, honey, orange juice, coconut oil, and vanilla in a bowl. **2** In a separate bowl, mix the almond flour, cinnamon, baking soda, and salt. **3** Using a rubber spatula, mix the wet ingredients and dry ingredients until just combined. **4** Fill the prepared muffin tin with the batter, filling each cup ⅔ full. **5** Bake until a toothpick inserted into the center comes out clean, about 20 minutes. **6** Set the pan on a wire rack to cool.

Per serving: Calories 234 (From Fat 157); Fat 18g (Saturated 6g); Cholesterol 37mg; Sodium 208mg; Carbohydrate 17g (Dietary Fiber 3g); Protein 6g.

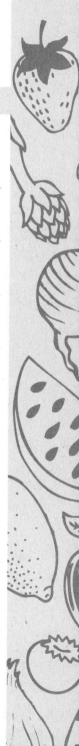

Chapter 11

Sauces, Fruit Spreads, and Nut Butters

In This Chapter

▶ Improving your cooking skills by making your own Paleo desserts

▶ Preparing delicious sweet Paleo condiments

*O*ne of the great things about living Paleo is that your cooking skills dramatically improve. Cooking foods from scratch is a wonderful skill to acquire, and it's one you must have to successfully live Paleo. You become more in tune with what you eat, how it's made, and what exactly is in it.

This chapter is dedicated to making a number of condiments that complement other dishes and treats. A little Chocolate Almond Butter turns any fruit into a decadent dessert. If chocolate isn't your thing, try the Truly Sugar-Free Strawberry Jam. It's great on ice cream, between two cookies, or spread on a piece of Paleo Sandwich Bread with some almond butter. (Check out Chapter 5 for the bread recipe).

Don't delay. Go whip up some delicious homemade jelly or a sweet caramel sauce — Paleo style! You'll be happy you did.

Truly Sugar-Free Strawberry Jam

Prep time: 10 min • **Cook time:** 50 min • **Yield:** 1 cup (11 servings)

Ingredients	Directions
2½ cups frozen strawberries, thawed	*1* Puree the strawberries in a food processor or blender.
1 tablespoon water	*2* Whisk the remaining ingredients in a medium saucepan and then mix in the strawberry puree.
1 tablespoon fresh lemon juice	
2 teaspoons arrowroot powder	*3* Bring mixture to a boil slowly over medium heat, stirring frequently.
	4 Lower the heat to medium low and simmer until the mixture thickens, approximately 50 minutes, stirring frequently to avoid burning. It's done when you can draw a channel through the center that stays open for a few seconds before filling in.
	5 Remove the mixture from the heat and allow it to cool before storing. As it cools, it will continue to thicken. Keep refrigerated in an airtight container.

Tip: You can use fresh strawberries in place of frozen ones. Heat 2½ cups fresh strawberries in a saucepan with the water, lemon juice, and arrowroot powder for 5 minutes over medium heat to soften the berries. Puree the mixture in your blender or food processor and then return the mixture to the saucepan and proceed with Step 3.

Tip: If your jam becomes too thick as it cools, add a little water. If it isn't thick enough, you can also return it to the stove and cook it longer (continuing to stir frequently so it doesn't burn).

Per serving/per tablespoon: Calories 10 (From Fat 0); Fat 0g (Saturated 0g); Cholesterol 0mg; Sodium 1mg; Carbohydrate 3g (Dietary Fiber 1g); Protein 0g.

Sugar-Free Blueberry Butter

Prep time: 15 min • **Cook time:** 25 min • **Yield:** 1 cup (11 servings)

Ingredients	Directions
2½ cups frozen blueberries, thawed	**1** Puree the blueberries in a food processor or blender.
1 tablespoon water	**2** Whisk the remaining ingredients in a medium saucepan and add the blueberry puree.
1 tablespoon fresh lemon juice	
1½ teaspoons arrowroot powder	**3** Bring the mixture to a boil slowly over medium heat, stirring frequently; simmer until it thickens, approximately 25 minutes. It's done when you can draw a channel through the center that stays open for a few seconds before filling in.
	4 Remove the pan from the heat. Process the mixture in the blender for a few seconds, or blend with a hand blender directly in the saucepan.
	5 Let the mixture cool. As it cools, it will continue to thicken. Keep refrigerated in an airtight container.

Tip: You can use fresh blueberries rather than frozen for this recipe. Heat 2½ cups of fresh blueberries in a saucepan with the water, lemon juice, and arrowroot powder for 5 minutes to soften the blueberries. Process the mixture in your blender or food processor and then return it to the stove and proceed with Step 3.

Tip: If your butter becomes too thick, add a little water. If you want it to be thicker, you can return it to the stove and cook it longer (stirring frequently).

Per serving/per tablespoon: Calories 14 (From Fat 1); Fat 0g (Saturated 0g); Cholesterol 0mg; Sodium 0mg; Carbohydrate 3g (Dietary Fiber 1g); Protein 0g.

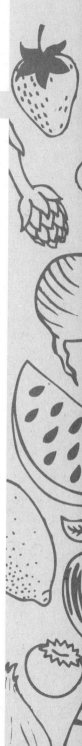

Chocolate Almond Butter

Prep time: 20 min • **Cook time:** 10 min • **Yield:** 1 cup (11 servings)

Ingredients	Directions
2 cups raw almonds	*1* Preheat the oven to 350 degrees.
1 tablespoon cacao butter	*2* Roast the almonds until they're fragrant and start to turn brown, about 10 minutes.
4½ tablespoons raw cacao powder	*3* Let the almonds cool for 5 minutes and then process them in a food processor or high-speed blender until smooth and creamy, scraping the sides of the bowl as needed. Using a spatula, mix in the cacao powder until combined.
1 tablespoon raw honey	
½ teaspoon vanilla extract	
1 tablespoon coconut oil, melted	
Pinch of salt	*4* Slowly melt the cacao butter in a bowl over simmering water (double boiler). Remove the bowl from the heat and mix in the honey, vanilla, coconut oil, and salt.
	5 Add the almond butter to the cacao mixture and mix to combine.
	6 Store in an airtight container in the fridge or at room temperature.

Per serving/per tablespoon: Calories 132 (From Fat 100); Fat 11g (Saturated 2g); Cholesterol 0mg; Sodium 10mg; Carbohydrate 6g (Dietary Fiber 3g); Protein 4g.

Homemade Chocolate Hazelnut Spread

Prep time: 20 min • **Yield:** 1 cup (11 servings)

Ingredients	Directions
3½ tablespoons Paleo-friendly 100% dark, unsweetened chocolate	**1** Melt the dark chocolate in a bowl over simmering water (double boiler).
1 cup hazelnut butter	**2** When the chocolate is melted, remove the bowl from heat and gently mix in the remaining ingredients with a rubber spatula.
1 tablespoon raw cacao powder	
2½ tablespoons raw honey, or to taste	**3** Store in an airtight glass jar in the fridge.
1 teaspoon vanilla extract	
Pinch of salt	
2 tablespoons coconut oil, melted	
6 tablespoons almond milk	

Tip: You can substitute your Paleo-friendly milk of choice — hazelnut milk, coconut milk, raw milk, or whatever you prefer — in Step 2.

Tip: You can save money and make your own hazelnut butter at home. Process 2¼ cups of blanched hazelnuts in a food processor or high-speed blender for a few minutes, scraping the sides of the bowl as needed until the nuts are creamy and smooth. If you can only find hazelnuts with the skin, roast them first 350 degrees until the skin begins to crack, about 10 minutes. Allow them to cool for 5 minutes, peel off the skins, and process the skinned hazelnuts in the food processor until creamy.

Tip: If you make your own hazelnut butter, stir all the ingredients together with a spatula in a bowl. Don't just pulse all the ingredients in the food processor, or the oils from the nuts will separate.

Vary It! Want an even faster version of this spread? Mix 1 cup hazelnut butter, 4 tablespoons raw cacao powder, ½ teaspoon vanilla extract, 1 tablespoon melted coconut oil, 3 tablespoons organic coconut palm sugar, and a pinch of salt with a rubber spatula. Store the mixture in an airtight glass jar in the fridge or at room temperature.

Per serving: Calories 365 (From Fat 280); Fat 31g (Saturated 9g); Cholesterol 0mg; Sodium 31mg; Carbohydrate 17g (Dietary Fiber 7g); Protein 9g.

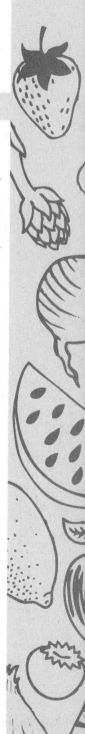

Coconut-Hazelnut Butter with Cacao Nibs

Prep time: 15 min • **Yield:** 1 cup (11 servings)

Ingredients	Directions
1 cup unsweetened shredded coconut **1 cup blanched hazelnuts** **¾ teaspoon vanilla extract** **3 tablespoons raw cacao nibs** **Pinch of salt**	*1* Pulse the coconut in a food processor or high-speed blender until creamy and liquid, scraping the sides of the bowl as needed. Repeat this process with the hazelnuts. *2* Combine the coconut butter and hazelnut butter in a glass jar and stir in the remaining ingredients. *3* Store at room temperature or in the fridge.

Tip: You can skip Step 1 and use ½ cup of store-bought coconut butter and ½ cup store-bought hazelnut butter in Step 2.

Tip: If you can only find hazelnuts with the skin, roast them first at 350 degrees until the skins begin to crack, about 10 minutes. Allow them to cool for 5 minutes, peel off the skins, and process the skinned hazelnuts in the food processor until creamy.

Per serving/per tablespoon; Calories 107 (From Fat 89); Fat 10g (Saturated 4g); Cholesterol 0mg; Sodium 10mg; Carbohydrate 3g (Dietary Fiber 2g); Protein 2g.

Caramel Sauce

Prep time: 5 min • **Cook time:** 15 min • **Yield:** ⅓ cup (11 servings)

Ingredients	Directions
2 tablespoons water	*1* Bring the water and coconut sugar to a boil over medium heat, stirring constantly.
¼ cup organic coconut palm sugar	
½ cup full-fat coconut milk	*2* Add the remaining ingredients and cook for about 10 minutes over medium heat, stirring constantly so that it doesn't burn. The mixture will start to thicken and turn darker.
1 teaspoon vanilla extract	
Pinch of salt	
	3 Store in an airtight container in the fridge.

Tip: The caramel thickens as it cools, but you can adjust its consistency. If you want it to be thicker, return it to the stove and cook it longer. For a thinner caramel sauce, add water 1 teaspoon at a time until the consistency is what you want.

Per serving/per tablespoon: Calories 96 (From Fat 36); Fat 4g (Saturated 3g); Cholesterol 0mg; Sodium 37mg; Carbohydrate 16g (Dietary Fiber 0g); Protein 0g.

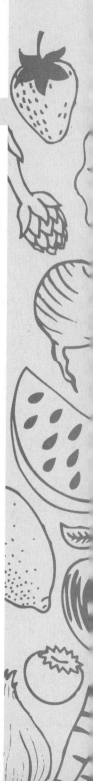

Dark Chocolate Fondue

Prep time: 5 min • **Cook time:** 5 min • **Yield:** 1 cup (11 servings)

Ingredients	Directions
6 tablespoons coconut oil, melted	**1** Place all the ingredients in a large heat-proof bowl. Set the bowl over a saucepan with a dash of water (double boiler) and simmer over low heat, making sure the water doesn't touch the bottom of the bowl.
4 tablespoons raw cacao powder	
2 tablespoons raw honey	**2** Stir until all the ingredients are combined and the mixture thickens.
6 tablespoons full-fat coconut milk	
2 teaspoons vanilla extract	**3** Serve immediately with fresh fruits or pour into an airtight container and store it in the fridge. Reheat the chocolate over a double boiler as needed.
1 tablespoon arrowroot powder	
Pinch of salt	

Per serving/per tablespoon (without fruit): Calories 74 (From Fat 57); Fat 7g (Saturated 6g); Cholesterol 0mg; Sodium 11mg; Carbohydrate 4g (Dietary Fiber 0g); Protein 1g.

Chocolate Fudge Ice Cream Topping

Prep time: 5 min • **Cook time:** 5 min • **Yield:** 1 cup (11 servings)

Ingredients	Directions
3½ tablespoons chopped Paleo-friendly 100% dark, unsweetened chocolate	*1* Melt the chocolate in a bowl over simmering water (double boiler).
1 tablespoon raw cacao powder	*2* After the chocolate has melted, stir in the remaining ingredients until thick, creamy, and smooth.
2½ tablespoons raw honey	
2½ tablespoons full-fat coconut milk	*3* Let the mixture cool for 5 minutes.
¼ teaspoon vanilla extract	*4* Pour the fudge immediately over ice cream or store it in an airtight container in the fridge. Reheat the fudge in a double boiler as needed.
Pinch of salt	

Per serving/per tablespoon: Calories 51 (From Fat 27); Fat 3g (Saturated 2g); Cholesterol 0mg; Sodium 20mg; Carbohydrate 7g (Dietary Fiber 1g); Protein 1g.

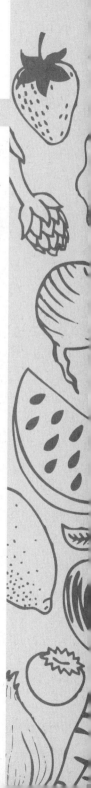

Part III
Sweet Holiday Paleo Desserts

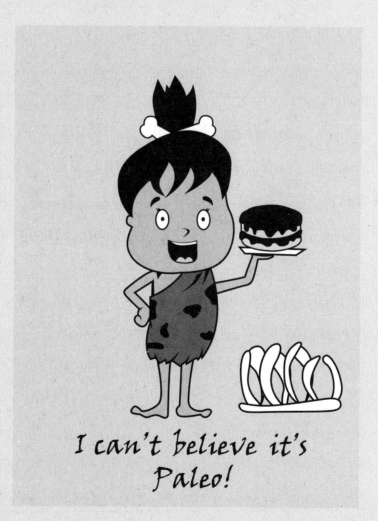

I can't believe it's Paleo!

In This Part . . .

✔ Enjoy a collection of healthy dessert recipes designed for holiday celebrations.

✔ Impress your holiday guests with desserts from pumpkin and apple pie to ginger cookies.

✔ Treat your friends and family to healthy treats without them feeling heavy and tired afterwards.

Chapter 12

Paleo Halloween

In This Chapter

▶ Keeping kids away from spooky toxic candy

▶ Creating homemade Paleo-ween treats

Recipes in This Chapter

▶ Ghost Truffles

▶ Raspberry Gummies

▶ Yummy Mummy Shortbread Cookies

▶ White Chocolate Pecan Butter Cups

*rick or treat! Celebrating Halloween can be difficult and worrisome for many Paleo parents. This holiday is when all the little monsters and witches head down the streets, knocking on doors and gathering bags of sugar-loaded, teeth-rotting, disease-causing candy. You want your children to enjoy being kids, but you also worry about the foods they're exposed to that may harm them. All of this franken-candy being passed around definitely makes for a frightening holiday.

As a Paleo parent, you can certainly keep the fun and the creepy factors of Halloween in your little ones' lives. Switch the focus from going out trick-or-treating to decorating the house, making costumes, carving pumpkins, hosting parties, or making your own healthful treats at home. Time spent cooking with your family in the kitchen is something you'll cherish for a lifetime, and your children will take great pride in their own culinary masterpieces!

This chapter gives you a selection of healthier treat alternatives that are spooky, cute, and fun — perfect for serving and sharing with kids at your Paleo-ween party!

Ghost Truffles

Prep time: 25 min, plus freezing time • **Yield:** 11 servings

Ingredients	Directions
3 tablespoons cacao paste	**1** Melt the cacao paste slowly in a bowl over simmering water (double boiler).
⅔ cup raw pecans, finely chopped	
½ cup melted coconut butter, divided	**2** Mix in the pecans, 4 tablespoons of the coconut butter, the honey, the vanilla, and the salt until well combined.
2 tablespoons raw honey (or more to taste)	**3** Scoop tablespoonfuls of dough onto a cookie sheet lined with parchment paper. Using your hands, shape each truffle into a 1-inch ball. The batter will be slightly crumbly, so shape each truffle gently and set it on the pan.
½ teaspoon vanilla extract	
Pinch of salt	
½ cup unsweetened shredded coconut	**4** Insert a lollipop stick into the center of each truffle and freeze for 20 minutes.
2 tablespoons of Paleo-friendly mini chocolate chips	**5** Dip the chilled truffles one at a time in the remaining coconut butter and then roll them in the shredded coconut. Return them to the sheet.
	6 Press three chocolate chips into each truffle to create a cute face. Keep refrigerated (the coconut butter melts at temperatures above 72 degrees).

Tip: To melt the coconut butter, place the jar in a large bowl of hot water. Stir the contents in the jar before using.

Vary It! In place of cacao paste you can use 100-percent unsweetened dark chocolate. Coarsely chop the cacao paste or unsweetened chocolate and measure your tablespoons.

Per serving: Calories 256 (From Fat 205); Fat 23g (Saturated 13g); Cholesterol 0mg; Sodium 17mg; Carbohydrate 13g (Dietary Fiber 2g); Protein 2g.

Raspberry Gummies

Prep time: 25 min, plus chilling time • **Cook time:** 5 min • **Yield:** 10 servings

Ingredients	Directions
1 cup raspberries, fresh or frozen and thawed	*1* Pulse the raspberries in a food processor or blender until smooth.
½ cup fresh lemon juice	*2* Pour the raspberry puree into a strainer set over a bowl and gently press the berries to extract the raspberry juice.
6 tablespoons unflavored powdered grass-fed gelatin	
2 tablespoons raw honey	*3* In a saucepan, whisk ¼ cup of the raspberry juice, the lemon juice, gelatin, and honey.
	4 Heat the mixture slowly over medium heat, stirring constantly until the gelatin is melted and all ingredients are well combined.
	5 Pour the mixture carefully into Halloween-shaped silicon candy molds.
	6 Refrigerate until the gummies harden, about 1 hour.

Per serving: *Calories 35 (From Fat 0); Fat 0g (Saturated 0g); Cholesterol 0mg; Sodium 9mg; Carbohydrate 6g (Dietary Fiber 0g); Protein 4g.*

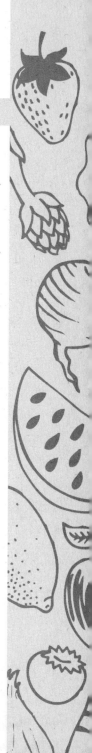

Yummy Mummy Shortbread Cookies

Prep time: 15 min • **Cook time:** 14 min • **Yield:** 14 servings

Ingredients	Directions

Ingredients

1¾ cup blanched almond flour

½ cup arrowroot powder

Pinch of salt

9 tablespoons coconut oil, melted and divided

4 tablespoons raw honey

1 tablespoon vanilla extract

⅔ cup Paleo-friendly dark chocolate, chopped

28 Paleo-friendly mini chocolate chips, divided

14 sliced cashews or almonds

Directions

1 Preheat the oven to 325 degrees and line a cookie sheet with parchment paper.

2 Mix the almond flour, arrowroot powder, and salt in a bowl.

3 In a separate bowl, whisk together 8 tablespoons of the coconut oil, the honey, and the vanilla. Using a rubber spatula, mix the wet ingredients and dry ingredients until just combined. Don't overmix.

4 Using your hands and about 1½ tablespoons per cookie, shape the dough into a 3x1.5-inch logs. Put logs on cookie sheet.

5 Freeze the cookie sheet for 5 minutes and then bake until the bottom and edges of the cookies start to turn brown, about 14 minutes. Place the cookie sheet on a wire rack to cool. Allow cookies to cool completely before dipping each cooking in chocolate (see Step 7).

6 Melt half of the dark chocolate in a bowl over simmering water (double boiler). Remove the bowl from the heat and slowly stir in the remaining dark chocolate and coconut oil until melted.

7 To create a mummy look, dip the tip of one end of each cookie in the melted chocolate; then dip the other end halfway in the chocolate, leaving a small space without chocolate. Set the cookies back on the cookie sheet with parchment paper.

8 Coat the back of two mini chocolate chips with melted chocolate and then place them in the white part of the cookie to make the mummy's eyes. Add a cashew or an almond below the eyes to form the mouth.

Tip: You can further decorate each cookie however you like.

Per serving: Calories 301 (From Fat 211); Fat 24g (Saturated 12g); Cholesterol 0mg; Sodium 16mg; Carbohydrate 23g (Dietary Fiber 4g); Protein 5g.

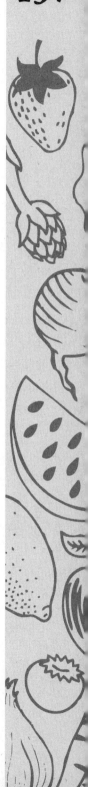

White Chocolate Pecan Butter Cups

Prep time: 20 min, plus freezing time • **Yield:** 7 servings

Ingredients	Directions
½ **cup shaved cacao butter**	**1** Melt the cacao butter slowly in a bowl over simmering water (double boiler).
½ **cup macadamia nuts**	
1 teaspoon vanilla extract	**2** Process the melted cacao butter, macadamia nuts, vanilla, honey, and salt in a food processor until creamy and liquidy, scraping the sides of the bowl as needed.
1 tablespoon raw honey	
Pinch of salt	
1 cup raw pecans	
	3 Pour two teaspoons of the cacao mixture into seven silicon baking cups and freeze until hardened, about 30 minutes.
	4 Meanwhile, process the pecans in a food processor until a creamy, smooth butter forms.
	5 Remove the cups from the freezer and add one teaspoon of the pecan butter to the center. Return to the freezer for 10 minutes.
	6 Remove the cups from the freezer and top with two teaspoons of the cacao mixture; freeze until hardened.
	7 Store the cups in an airtight container in the fridge or freezer. These cups melt at room temperature.

Tip: You can use store-bought pecan butter instead of making your own. Just omit the pecans, skip Step 4, and start with ¼ cup pecan butter in Step 5.

Vary It! Sweetening the cacao mixture with 3 tablespoons of organic coconut palm sugar rather than the honey will make the taste better resemble that of traditional white chocolate. However, the color of your chocolate may be darker.

Per serving: Calories 322 (From Fat 302); Fat 34g (Saturated 12g); Cholesterol 0mg; Sodium 23mg; Carbohydrate 6g (Dietary Fiber 2g); Protein 2g.

Chapter 13

Paleo Thanksgiving

In This Chapter

▶ Giving thanks for healthful food

▶ Celebrating Thanksgiving with Paleo desserts

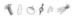
Gobble, gobble, gobble! As the holiday season approaches, food becomes a major part of family gatherings, work parties, and social events. Thanksgiving is a time when families and friends reunite to give thanks for a whole year's worth of blessings, often by sharing a meal.

Preparing Paleo desserts for the Thanksgiving spread is a perfect way to help balance out the table and show your loved ones all the creative ways they can incorporate healthy foods into the holiday feast. It's a perfect time of year to help people enjoy wonderful foods without all the post-meal, bogged-down blues.

The recipes in this chapter let you make your next Thanksgiving one to remember with delicious, mouthwatering Paleo fall staple desserts. Your guests will be blown away, and everyone will be able to go home feeling guilt-free!

Marble Pumpkin Bread

Prep time: 20 min • **Cook time:** 40 min • **Yield:** 15 servings

Ingredients	Directions
1 cup organic canned pumpkin puree	*1* Preheat the oven to 350 degrees.
2 tablespoons coconut cream	*2* In a large bowl, whisk the pumpkin puree, coconut cream, coconut oil, eggs, vanilla, and honey.
3 tablespoons coconut oil, melted	
2 room temperature eggs	*3* In a separate bowl, mix the almond flour, baking soda, salt, flaxseed meal and cinnamon. Chop the pecans in a food processor and mix them with the almond flour mixture.
1 teaspoon vanilla extract	
⅓ cup raw honey	
2 cups blanched almond flour	*4* Using a rubber spatula, gently mix the dry ingredients and wet ingredients together. Don't overmix. The batter will be thick.
1 teaspoon baking soda	
½ teaspoon salt	
2 tablespoons flaxseed meal	*5* Reserve 2 cups of the batter and pour the remaining batter in an 8½-x-4½-inch medium loaf pan lined with parchment paper.
1½ teaspoons ground cinnamon	
½ cup pecans	*6* Mix the cacao powder into 1 cup of the reserved batter. Evenly spread this mixture on top of the batter in the pan.
¼ cup raw cacao powder	
⅓ cup Paleo-friendly chocolate chunks	*7* Top the chocolate batter layer with the remaining cup of reserved batter and gently swirl all the layers together with a knife. Don't overswirl, or you'll end up with an all-chocolate batter.

8 Sprinkle the top of the loaf with the chocolate chunks and bake until a toothpick inserted into the center comes out clean, approximately 40 minutes.

9 Set the pan on a wire rack to cool. To preserve freshness, wrap the loaf in paper towel and store it in an airtight container in the refrigerator.

Tip: Coconut cream is the thick cream that forms on the top of a can of full-fat coconut milk when you leave it in the fridge overnight, discarding the water.

Per serving: Calories 229 (From Fat 161); Fat 18g (Saturated 6g); Cholesterol 25mg; Sodium 177mg; Carbohydrate 17g (Dietary Fiber 5g); Protein 6g.

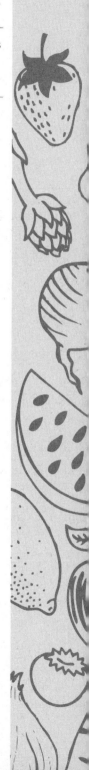

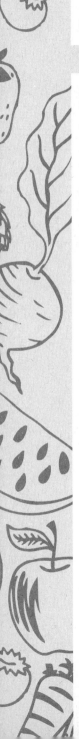

No-Bake Triple Chocolate Pumpkin Pie

Prep time: 20 min, plus chilling time • **Yield:** 15 servings

Ingredients	Directions
Chocolate Pumpkin Filling (see the following recipe)	**1** Grease a 9-inch removable-bottom tart pan with coconut oil and place a piece of parchment paper on the bottom of the pan.
1½ cups raw pecans	
1 cup Medjool dates (about 10–12 large dates), pitted	**2** Chop the pecans in a food processor until they form a coarse meal; remove them to a large bowl.
4 tablespoons raw cacao powder	**3** Process the dates in the food processor until a creamy paste forms. Using your hands, mix the chopped pecans, date paste, and raw cacao powder. Press the crust mixture onto the bottom and sides of the prepared tart pan.
¼ cup Paleo-friendly chocolate chips, melted	
	4 Evenly pour the Chocolate Pumpkin Filling over the crust.
	5 Melt the chocolate chips slowly in a large bowl over simmering water (double boiler) and drizzle the chocolate over the pie. Refrigerate until the pie is set, about 4 hours.

Chocolate Pumpkin Filling

2 ounces 100-percent Paleo-friendly dark, unsweetened chocolate

One 15-ounce organic can pumpkin puree

4 tablespoons raw honey

3 tablespoons coconut oil, melted

¼ teaspoon ground cinnamon

Generous pinch of salt

1 Melt the chocolate slowly in a large bowl over simmering water (double boiler).

2 When the chocolate is melted, remove the bowl from the heat and add the pumpkin puree, honey, coconut oil, cinnamon, and salt.

3 Using a rubber spatula, mix until all ingredients are combined.

Per serving: Calories 306 (From Fat 185); Fat 21g (Saturated 8g); Cholesterol 0mg; Sodium 22mg; Carbohydrate 34g (Dietary Fiber 7g); Protein 4g.

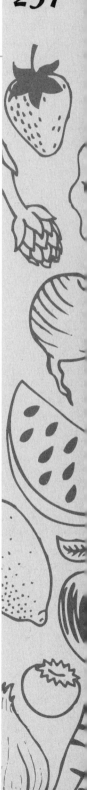

Fudgy Pumpkin Blondies with Dark Chocolate Chunks

Prep time: 15 min • **Cook time:** 25 min • **Yield:** 10 servings

Ingredients	Directions
2 cups blanched almond flour ½ cup flaxseed meal 2 teaspoons ground cinnamon ½ cup organic coconut palm sugar ½ teaspoon salt 1 egg 1 cup organic canned pumpkin puree 1 tablespoon vanilla extract 1 tablespoon raw honey ⅓ cup Paleo-friendly chocolate chunks	*1* Preheat the oven to 350 degrees and line an 8-inch square pan with parchment paper, covering all four sides of the pan. *2* Mix the almond flour, flaxseed meal, cinnamon, coconut sugar, and salt in a bowl. *3* In a separate bowl, whisk the egg, pumpkin puree, vanilla, and honey. *4* Using a rubber spatula, gently mix the dry ingredients and wet ingredients together. Don't overmix. Fold the chocolate chunks into the batter. Spoon the batter evenly into the prepared baking pan. *5* Bake until a toothpick inserted into the center comes out clean, approximately 25 minutes. *6* Set the pan over a wire rack to cool and then cut the blondies into 2-inch squares. Store in the fridge.

Tip: After you pour the batter into the pan, top it with a few extra chocolate chunks.

Tip: Use chocolate chunks by Enjoy Life brand which are nut-, dairy-, and soy-free. Alternatively, you can chop any Paleo-friendly chocolate bar into large pieces to use in this recipe.

Per serving: Calories 265 (From Fat 146); Fat 16g (Saturated 3g); Cholesterol 19mg; Sodium 137mg; Carbohydrate 26g (Dietary Fiber 6g); Protein 8g.

No-Bake Carrot Cake Truffles

Prep time: 20 min, plus chilling time • **Yield:** 15 servings

Ingredients	Directions
4 large Medjool dates, pitted	**1** Process the dates in a food processor until creamy. Add the carrots, almond flour, pecans, flaxseed meal, vanilla, cinnamon, and salt and pulse until everything is combined.
1 cup finely grated carrots	
½ cup blanched almond flour	
½ cup pecans, coarsely chopped	**2** Roll the mixture into balls (about 1½ teaspoons per ball) and place them on a baking sheet lined with parchment paper. Place the sheet in the freezer.
1 tablespoon flaxseed meal	
2 teaspoons vanilla extract	
⅛ teaspoon cinnamon	**3** Slowly melt half the chocolate in a bowl over simmering water (double boiler).
⅛ teaspoon salt	
⅓ cup plus 1 tablespoon dark chocolate, chopped	**4** Remove the bowl from the stove and stir in the other half of the chocolate and the coconut oil until smooth.
1 teaspoon coconut oil, melted	
	5 Dip the chilled carrot cake truffles in the chocolate and set them back on the parchment paper.
	6 Chill the truffles in the refrigerator until the chocolate hardens. Keep refrigerated.

Per serving: Calories 95 (From Fat 59); Fat 7g (Saturated 2g); Cholesterol 0mg; Sodium 28mg; Carbohydrate 8g (Dietary Fiber 2g); Protein 2g.

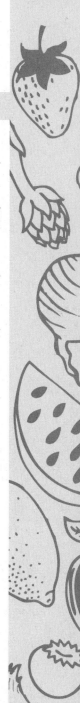

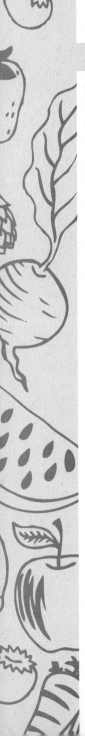

Chocolate Pecan Pie Bars

Prep time: 25 min, plus chilling time • **Cook time:** 24 min • **Yield:** 10 servings

Ingredients	Directions
Chocolate Pecan Filling (see the following recipe) ½ cup pecans, coarsely chopped 6 tablespoons pastured butter, melted 1 tablespoon raw honey 1 cup blanched almond flour ½ cup Paleo-friendly dark chocolate, chopped ½ cup whole raw pecans	**1** Preheat the oven to 350 degrees and line an 8-x-8-inch baking pan with parchment paper, covering all four sides of the pan. **2** Using a rubber spatula, mix the chopped pecans, butter, honey, and almond flour in a bowl. **3** Spread the mixture evenly on the bottom of the prepared baking pan. Bake for 12 minutes or until the top starts to brown. Set the pan on a wire rack to cool. **4** Pour the Chocolate Pecan Filling over the baked crust and return it to the oven for about 12 minutes or until the filling is set. Set the pan on a wire rack to cool. **5** Melt the dark chocolate in a bowl over simmering water (double boiler) and then pour it evenly over the top of the pie. Sprinkle the pie with whole pecans. **6** Refrigerate the pie for 15 minutes and then cut it into squares.

Chocolate Pecan Filling

5 tablespoons room temperature water

2 tablespoons pastured butter, melted

¼ cup raw cacao powder

3 tablespoons raw honey

1 teaspoon vanilla extract

2 room temperature eggs

Pinch of salt

1 Whisk all the ingredients in a bowl.

Vary It! You can use *ghee* (clarified butter) or coconut oil in place of the pastured butter in both the crust and the filling.

Per serving: Calories 320(From Fat 244); Fat 27g (Saturated 10g); Cholesterol 62mg; Sodium 80mg; Carbohydrate 14g (Dietary Fiber 4g); Protein 6g.

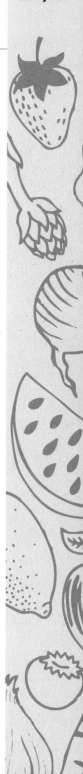

Chapter 14

Paleo Christmas and Hanukkah

In This Chapter

▶ Enjoying the holiday season without setbacks

▶ Sharing a collection Paleo Christmas and Hanukkah sweets

As soon as you've made it through the Thanksgiving holiday, Christmas and Hanukkah pop up, and you're back at the dinner table again! Whether it's festive lunches at the office, dinners with family, or the constant barrage of desserts and snacks everywhere you go, you have to do your best not to fall into a food coma.

If you're just now transitioning to eating nutrient-dense foods on the Paleo diet, the holidays are the perfect time to start making a new and improved nutritious menu to share with your family and friends. Try incorporating some Paleo-friendly sides, veggies, and, of course, condiments and desserts. (For a wide range of non-dessert Paleo recipes, check out *Paleo Cookbook For Dummies* by Kellyann Petrucci [Wiley].)

I love the holiday season, especially because I get to share with others how to have delicious, healthy, and nourishing sweets when you're surrounded by so many unhealthy choices. In this chapter, I show you how to make a handful of Paleo dessert recipes geared toward Christmas and Hanukkah. Making your own treats helps you stay on your healthy Paleo path and not fall for unhealthy temptations during this festive season.

Chocolate Pinwheel Cookies

Prep time: 1 hr, plus freezing time • **Cook time:** 10 min • **Yield:** 20 servings

Ingredients	Directions
¼ cup Paleo-friendly chocolate chips	*1* Preheat the oven to 325 degrees and line a cookie sheet with parchment paper.
2 cups blanched almond flour	
2 tablespoons arrowroot powder	*2* Melt the chocolate chips in a bowl over simmering water (double boiler). Set aside.
½ teaspoon salt	
5 tablespoons pastured butter, softened	*3* Mix the almond flour, arrowroot powder, and salt in a bowl.
2 large room temperature egg yolks	*4* In a separate bowl, whisk the butter, egg yolks, honey and vanilla. Using a rubber spatula, gently mix the dry ingredients and wet ingredients together, being careful to not overmix.
3 tablespoons raw honey	
2 teaspoons vanilla extract	
2 tablespoons raw cacao powder	*5* Shape half of the dough into a ball and set aside. To the remaining dough, add the cacao powder and melted chocolate and mix gently but thoroughly. Then shape the chocolate dough into a ball.
	6 Press each dough into a disk and then wrap each dough disk separately in plastic wrap. Freeze for 30 minutes.
	7 Roll the vanilla dough into a 10-inch square between two pieces of parchment paper.
	8 Repeat the process with the chocolate dough, using fresh parchment, and then remove the top sheet of parchment from each square.

9 Flip the chocolate dough on top of the vanilla dough. Gently roll over the top with a rolling pin to make the dough pieces adhere to each other.

10 Trim the edges of the dough with a knife and then carefully roll the dough into a tight log. If you have trouble rolling the log, lift up the parchment paper and use it for leverage.

11 Freeze the dough for 30 minutes.

12 Cut the chilled dough into ¼-inch-thick cookies and transfer each piece to the prepared cookie sheet. Bake for about 10 minutes, or until the top and edges start to turn brown.

13 Allow the cookies to cool on the baking sheet for 5 minutes and then transfer them to a wire rack.

Per serving: Calories 128 (From Fat 91); Fat 10g (Saturated 3g); Cholesterol 26mg; Sodium 64mg; Carbohydrate 8g (Dietary Fiber 2g); Protein 3g.

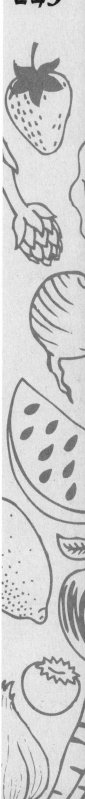

Chocolate Hazelnut Thumbprint Cookies

Prep time: 25 min • **Cook time:** 10–12 min • **Yield:** 14 servings

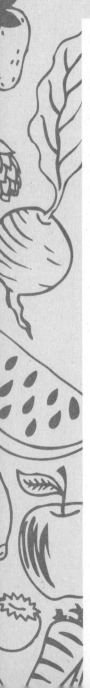

Ingredients	Directions
⅓ cup whole blanched hazelnuts	**1** Preheat the oven to 350 degrees and line a cookie sheet with parchment paper.
¾ cup blanched almond flour	
4 tablespoons raw cacao powder	**2** Pulse the whole hazelnuts in a food processor until finely ground. In a large bowl, mix the ground hazelnuts, almond flour, cacao powder, baking soda, and salt.
½ teaspoon baking soda	
Pinch of salt	
3 tablespoons coconut oil, melted	**3** In a separate bowl, whisk the coconut oil, honey, and hazelnut extract. Using a rubber spatula, mix the dry ingredients and wet ingredients together just until combined.
2 tablespoons raw honey	
1 teaspoon hazelnut extract	
½ cup blanched hazelnuts, coarsely chopped (optional)	**4** Shape the dough into 1-inch balls and then roll each ball in the chopped hazelnuts (if desired).
¼ cup Paleo-friendly chocolate chips	**5** Place the balls on the prepared cookie sheet and make an indentation in the center of each ball with your thumb.
1 tablespoon coconut cream	
	6 Bake for 10 to 12 minutes. Immediately upon removal, press down the center of each cookie (careful, they'll be hot) and set the cookie sheet on a wire rack to cool.

7 Melt the chocolate chips slowly in a bowl over simmering water (double boiler). Stir in the coconut cream until smooth.

8 Spoon or pipe the chocolate into the center of each cookie and serve.

Tip: If you can't find blanched hazelnuts, purchase hazelnuts with the skin on. Roast them in the oven for a few minutes at 300 degrees, being careful not to burn. When the skin starts to crack, remove the nuts from the oven. Let them cool a bit; while they're still warm, peel off the skin.

Tip: Coconut cream is the cream that forms on the top of a can of full-fat coconut milk when you leave it in the fridge overnight, discarding the water.

Vary It! You can use vanilla extract in place of the hazelnut extract in Step 3. You can also substitute pastured butter for the coconut cream in Step 7.

Per serving: Calories 126 (From Fat 91); Fat 10g (Saturated 5g); Cholesterol 0mg; Sodium 0mg; Carbohydrate 8g (Dietary Fiber 2g); Protein 3g.

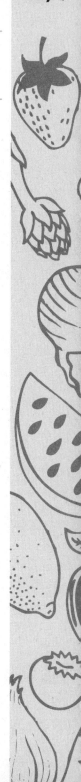

Peppermint Bark

Prep time: 20 min, plus chilling time • **Yield:** 15 servings

Ingredients	Directions
¾ cup Paleo-friendly dark chocolate chips	**1** Melt the chocolate chips in a bowl over simmering water (double boiler).
½ teaspoon peppermint extract	
2 tablespoons full-fat coconut milk	**2** Mix the peppermint extract and coconut milk into the melted chocolate until smooth. If your chocolate becomes thick, add 1 tablespoon of coconut oil at a time until you achieve the desired consistency.
¾ cup melted coconut butter	
⅓ cup fresh cranberries, chopped	**3** Line a 9-x-9-inch or 8-x-8-inch square pan with a large piece of parchment paper, covering the bottom and all four sides of the pan.
	4 Spread the chocolate evenly across the bottom of the pan and then freeze or refrigerate until the chocolate sets.
	5 Pour the melted coconut butter evenly over the top of chocolate and refrigerate for 5 minutes.
	6 Sprinkle with the chopped cranberries and refrigerate until the coconut layer is firm.
	7 Break or cut into small pieces and serve. Keep refrigerated.

Tip: To melt the coconut butter, place the glass jar in a pan of hot water. Stir the contents in the jar before using.

Vary It! You can use dried cranberries in place of the fresh fruit. Dried cranberries are usually dried with sugar and vegetable oils added. When you purchase dried cranberries, look for brands that list cranberries as the only ingredient, or use those that are sweetened with fruit juice.

Per serving: Calories 136 (From Fat 111); Fat 12g (Saturated 10g); Cholesterol 0mg; Sodium 5mg; Carbohydrate 10g (Dietary Fiber 4g); Protein 2g.

Soft and Chewy Ginger Cookies

Prep time: 15 min, plus freezing time • **Cook time:** 10 min • **Yield:** 22 servings

Ingredients	Directions
2⅔ cups blanched almond flour ½ cup organic coconut palm sugar 2 teaspoons ground ginger 1 teaspoon baking soda ½ teaspoon ground cinnamon ½ teaspoon ground nutmeg ¼ teaspoon salt 6 tablespoons pastured butter, softened 3 tablespoons raw honey 2 tablespoons water 1 egg	**1** In a large bowl, mix the almond flour, coconut sugar, ginger, baking soda, cinnamon, nutmeg, and salt. **2** In a separate bowl, beat the butter, honey, and water with an electric handheld or stand mixer until ingredients are combined. Then beat in the egg until everything is combined. **3** Using a rubber spatula, mix the dry and wet ingredients together. Don't overmix. Cover and freeze the dough for 1 hour or until it's easy to handle. **4** Preheat the oven to 350 degrees, and line a cookie sheet with parchment paper. **5** Roll the chilled dough into balls (about 1½ tablespoons per ball) and place them 2 inches apart on the prepared cookie sheet. Flatten each cookie slightly with the palm of your hand. **6** Bake for about 10 minutes or until the bottom and edges start to turn brown. **7** Set the baking sheet on a wire rack to cool.

Per serving: Calories 152 (From Fat 100); Fat 11g (Saturated 3g); Cholesterol 19mg; Sodium 104mg; Carbohydrate 12g (Dietary Fiber 2g); Protein 4g.

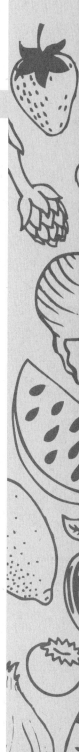

Paleo Apple Pie

Prep time: 1 hr • **Cook time:** 1 hr • **Yield:** 10 servings

Ingredients	Directions
Almond Flour Crust (see the following recipe)	*1* Preheat the oven to 400 degrees.
Streusel Topping (see the following recipe)	*2* In a large bowl, combine the apples, lime juice, coconut oil, and cinnamon.
4 to 5 medium apples, peeled, cored, and sliced to ¼-inch thickness	*3* In a medium saucepan, stir the coconut sugar and water. Heat the mixture over medium heat until the sugar dissolves. Mix in the coconut milk and simmer for 10 minutes, stirring constantly, to form a caramel.
1 tablespoon fresh lime juice	
2 tablespoons coconut oil, melted	*4* Remove the caramel from the heat and pour it over the apples. Toss until the apples are fully coated.
1 teaspoon ground cinnamon	
⅓ cup organic coconut palm sugar	*5* Spoon the apple filling over the chilled Almond Flour Crust and then distribute the Streusel Topping over the apples.
2 tablespoons water	
½ cup full-fat coconut milk	*6* Bake the pie for 10 minutes at 400 degrees. Reduce the temperature to 325 degrees and cover the pie with aluminum foil. Bake for another 40 minutes or until the apples are tender.
	7 Cool the pie completely on a wire rack. Serve warm or at room temperature.

Almond Flour Crust

2 cups blanched almond flour

½ cup coconut oil, melted

2 tablespoons cold full-fat coconut milk

2 tablespoons raw honey

1 Using a rubber spatula, mix all ingredients until just combined. Don't overmix.

2 Press the dough into the bottom and sides of a 9-inch glass pie dish. Create fluted edges with your fingers if desired (I like using gloves when working with this dough).

3 Cover the crust with plastic wrap or tin foil and freeze until you're ready to use it.

Streusel Topping

½ cup blanched almond flour

1 tablespoon plus 1 ½ teaspoons flaxseed meal

2 tablespoons arrowroot powder

2 tablespoons organic coconut palm sugar

1½ tablespoons coconut oil, melted

1½ teaspoons full-fat coconut milk

½ teaspoon vanilla extract

⅓ cup walnuts or pecans, coarsely chopped

1 Mix all ingredients with your hands. The mixture will be crumbly.

Tip: Using tart Granny Smith apples works well with this recipe because the caramel is very sweet. Also using a mixture of different types of apples adds to the texture of your pie; some stay firm, and some soften while baking.

Tip: Bake the crust for 9 minutes prior to adding the apple filling.

Per serving: Calories 457 (From Fat 324); Fat 37g (Saturated 17g); Cholesterol 0mg; Sodium 19mg; Carbohydrate 32g (Dietary Fiber 5g); Protein 8g.

Part IV
Part of Tens

the
part of
tens

In This Part . . .

✔ Learn tips and shortcuts to make your dessert creation a little easier.

✔ Discover how to make ingredient substitutions so your desserts are as yummy and healthy as possible.

Chapter 15

Ten Tips for Making Paleo Desserts

In This Chapter

▶ Starting your recipe off on the right foot

▶ Taking advantage of some tricks of the Paleo baking trade

C reating Paleo dessert recipes takes a lot of trial and error to get the final product to have just the right texture and flavor. Baking is a science, and learning the physical properties of cooking and the way Paleo ingredients behave together takes time and practice. I've spent a lot of time figuring out what works and what doesn't, and I'm here to share what I've learned: my best baking tips and advice.

In this chapter, I offer some additional tips and tricks that not only help you successfully recreate the recipes from this cookbook but also give you the tools to be creative in the kitchen and start developing your own recipes. Soon you'll be making delicious, healthy sweets that all your family and friends will be raving about.

Read the Recipe and Follow It Closely

Before you begin making a recipe, read through the ingredients list and the instructions carefully. Believe it or not, this step is the first and most important step to successfully bake that savory chocolate brownie you've been dreaming of.

Read the recipe from start to end. Make a list of the ingredients and go through your pantry to ensure you have everything. Run to the store to get what you're missing if necessary. *Remember:* Using the exact ingredients called for in a recipe is always better than making substitutions, especially the first time you try that recipe.

Finally, follow the instructions in order. Changing the order in which you mix the ingredients or the preparation method can sometimes make a big difference. For example, say a recipe for chocolate almond butter calls for mixing the chocolate with the almond butter with a spoon rather than with a food processor. If you don't follow that direction as written and use the food processor anyway, the oils in the butter will separate, and you'll end up with a thick, oily paste rather than a smooth, creamy butter.

Don't Overmix When Using Almond Flour

Overmixing with coconut flour or most other gluten-free flours isn't a problem, but that's not the case with almond flour. Almond flour is higher in fat than other flours, so the more you mix desserts made with almond flour, the more oil leaches out, and the more likely your product is to be dense, oily, or too moist. This is particularly important if you're using homemade almond flour that you grind yourself because homemade flour is usually much more moist than store-bought flour.

Use a wooden spoon or rubber spatula when mixing batter or dough made with almond flour. Stir just until the flour is incorporated into the mixture. If your batter is too wet, adding a small amount of coconut flour or starch such as tapioca or arrowroot powder to your recipe can help absorb the extra moistness.

Use a Combination of Flours, Starches, and Seeds

If you find yourself wanting to experiment with Paleo baked goods, use a combination of nut (or seed) flours and starches to replace wheat flours. Using a blend of starches with grain-free flours enhances the texture of baked goods, mimicking the structure and tenderness of flours that contain gluten. Adding 1 tablespoon of arrowroot powder to 2 cups of almond flour creates fluffy, tender crumbs in baked goods. You can add ¼ cup of arrowroot powder to ⅓ cup of coconut flour to achieve the same results.

Adding flaxseeds or flaxseed meal to breads, muffins, and cookies replicates the flavor of wheat-based flours. Ground flaxseeds and chia seeds also help bind ingredients together and recreate the elastic properties of gluten flours, cutting down on how many eggs you have to use

When you're baking cookies made with nut or seed flours and you want them to have a chewy texture with slightly crispy edges, bake them on a light-colored metal cookie sheet. On the other hand, if you want your cookies to be thin and crispy, bake them on a dark-colored cookie sheet. Using dark-colored pans also results in your cookies having a darker color.

Bring Ingredients to Room Temperature

You may have noticed that many recipes call for bringing ingredients to room temperature before mixing. That's because eggs, butter, milk, and other ingredients mix together more easily at room temperature (between 65 degrees and 70 degrees Fahrenheit). Using room temperature ingredients allows the batter to trap air, giving baked goods rise and creating light, tender crumbs.

The temperature of various ingredients also affects how other ingredients behave. For example, if you mix melted coconut oil with cold eggs, the coconut oil will start to solidify, and it won't mix properly and evenly with the other ingredients.

Allow your ingredients to come to room temperature on the countertop for about 30 minutes before using. To quickly bring eggs to room temperature, place them in a cup with warm water for 5 minutes. I often heat a cold can of coconut milk by placing the can in a pot of warm water and heating it over low heat for a few minutes.

Adjust the Sweetness of Your Recipes

No two dessert lovers have quite the same palate, so you may find some recipes too savory or too sweet for your taste. You can usually make some additions or substitutions to tweak the sweetness of your dish without breaking out the sugar. For instance, vanilla extract tastes wonderful and is sweet. Adding more vanilla to your recipe may just give it that extra sweetness you're looking for. Another great way to naturally sweeten your desserts is by adding a handful of fresh fruits such as berries, apple, banana, or mango. Dried fruits can also provide more sweetness, but keep in mind that dried fruits are sweeter than fresh fruits, so you don't need to add much. (And be sure they have no sugar or vegetable oils added.)

One sweetening option you may not be familiar with is lucuma powder. *Lucuma powder* is a low-glycemic sweetener made from the lucuma fruit, which is native to Peru and offers a rich source of beta carotene, iron, zinc, vitamin B3, calcium, and protein. The fruit is dried at low temperatures, preserving its natural vitamins and minerals, and then milled into fine powder. The powder makes a wonderful complement to other sweeteners with its sweet maple or caramel-like flavor.

If you want to reduce the sweetness and sugar content of your desserts when a recipe calls for chocolate chips (which are usually 50 to 70 percent dark), you can substitute half of the chocolate with chopped 100 percent dark, unsweetened baking chocolate. The finished product will still have that lovely chocolaty flavor.

As time goes by and your body adjusts to eating Paleo foods, your taste buds also change, and you begin to detect sweet flavors in nuts and even some vegetables, like broccoli. Soon you'll find that a little sweetener is all you need to make Paleo desserts sweet and flavorful.

Make Sure the Oven Is the Correct Temperature

Preheating your oven and ensuring it's heated to the correct temperature is essential for baking Paleo desserts to perfection. Set your oven to the desired temperature and allow it to warm up for at least 15 minutes before baking. For best results, don't rely on the oven's preheat sensor; I recommend purchasing an oven thermometer so you can confirm the oven has reached the correct temperature. You can find this cheap, useful tool at any kitchen store.

Don't open the oven door during baking until it's time to check for doneness (see the following section). Allow your product to cook for the estimated time directed in the recipe instructions. Opening the door prematurely may affect the temperature, as well as cause your baked product to fall.

Test Baked Goods for Doneness

Sometimes figuring out when baked goods have cooked long enough is hard. Some cookie recipes, for example, say the cookies are done when the bottom and edges start to turn brown. But how can you tell if dark-colored cookies, such as double chocolate cookies, have baked to the correct coloring? One way is by smell. When you begin to smell your cookies baking, it's a sign they're close to being done. Test for doneness by nudging and lightly pressing them with a spatula. If the edges feel firm, that's a good indication your cookies are done baking. You may also notice a hint of brown around the edges of each cookie.

The best way to tell when brownies, breads, muffins, and cakes have cooked long enough is by inserting a stick into the center and making sure it comes out clean (with no batter sticking to it). If the top of the product appears to have cooked long enough but the inside is still underbaked, you may cover the pan with aluminum foil to prevent the top from burning. However, this step isn't necessary unless the recipe instructions direct you to do it.

Use Parchment Paper and Silicone Bakeware for Nonstick Baking

Parchment paper and silicone bakeware are the perfect nonstick solution that eliminates the need for greasing cake pans and cookie sheets. *Parchment paper,* also known as *baking paper* or *bakery paper,* is a heat- and moisture-resistant paper with a nonstick surface on both sides.

Don't confuse parchment paper with waxed paper. Unlike waxed paper, parchment paper is safe to use in the oven at temperatures up to 420 to 450 degrees Fahrenheit, depending on the brand. However, you shouldn't use parchment paper to cook under a broiler.

Lining your baking pan with parchment paper saves you a mess, and it makes removing items from the pan quick and easy. You can cut the paper to fit into any pan size and use it more than once. Because nothing sticks to it, it's also great for rolling out doughs. Simply place the dough between two sheets of parchment paper and roll to the desired thickness with your rolling pin.

In some cases, you'll want to stop the paper from moving around in the baking pan. Coating the pan with a little bit of coconut or olive oil helps the paper stick to the pan.

Made of a stable synthetic material, silicone pans are heat resistant and provide a good nonstick alternative to using parchment paper. They eliminate the need for greasing the pan and can replace metal and other nonstick cookware. The pans are available in all shapes and sizes, and even come as flat sheets that you can line your cookie sheet with to bake perfect cookies without having to grease the pan. Silicone pans also freeze well and are great for molding gelatin, candy, and chocolate. Silicone baking pans are easy to clean with a little soap and water.

Chill Dough Before Rolling and Cutting

When making Paleo cookies, pastries, or pie crusts that require rolling the dough, freeze or refrigerate the dough until it's firm. Chilling the dough prior to rolling and cutting prevents it from being too sticky and makes it much easier to handle.

The best way to roll out Paleo doughs is by placing the chilled dough between two sheets of nonstick parchment paper or silicone mats and then rolling over it with a rolling pin or pressing down on it with a large, flat cutting board until your dough achieves the desired thickness.

If you're cutting out cookies, work with small amounts of dough at a time so that it's firm and easy to handle. Divide the dough in half and freeze each half wrapped separately in plastic wrap. Roll and cut cookies from one half of the dough, leaving the other in the freezer. Place the cut cookies in the fridge to keep them cold while you roll and cut the second half of the dough. If your dough becomes too soft and hard to handle at anytime, return it to the freezer until it's firm again.

Bake with the Finest Ingredients

Making Paleo desserts is very easy when you use the highest quality ingredients. Fresh organic fruits, eggs, and butter, as well as homemade coconut or nut milk (such as almond milk) gives your recipes the best results.

Make homemade milk using a blender by blending ½ cup of favorite nut or unsweetened shredded coconut with 2 cups of warm water for about 1 minute, and than strain the milk using a cheesecloth or fine mesh strainer.

Whether you're baking brownies or whipping up a fancy coconut whipped cream, the brand of ingredients you use also significantly affect the final texture and taste of your product. You don't need to be an experienced cook to make Paleo treats, and you don't need any fancy equipment, but using the recommended products is critical to success.

Recommended brands of blanched almond flour are by *Honeyville* and *Welbee's*; Organic full-fat coconut milk by *Thai Kitchen* has a wonderful flavor and optimal fat content; *Let's Do Organic Coconut Flour, Tropical Traditions,* and *Wilderness Family Naturals* are my suggested coconut flour brands; *Enjoy Life* carries dark chocolate chips and chunks that are soy, dairy, and nut free; *Earth Circle Organics* makes the most delicious raw cacao powder, and *Equal exchange* is my go to brand for soy-free, fairly traded organic dark chocolate.

Chapter 16

Ten Nutritious Paleo Food Substitutions

. . . .

In This Chapter

▶ Switching out non-Paleo ingredients

▶ Flooding your diet with better Paleo liquids

. . . .

*F*inding new alternatives to the foods that have been staples of your diet for so many years may be difficult as you transition to the Paleo diet. Luckily, you can replicate the texture and flavor of many of your favorite foods by using nutritious Paleo-friendly ingredients. Most of this book focuses on dessert alternatives (that's why it's called *Paleo Desserts For Dummies*), but because humans unfortunately can't live on dessert alone, this chapter looks at Paleo eating as a whole.

Substituting grains and other starches with veggies or swapping candy with savory sweets significantly boosts your daily intake of nutrients while satisfying any cravings you may have. Your Paleo approach to food and lifestyle also helps you become a better cook. Planning your meals in advance, shopping for local produce at farmers' markets, and using leftovers for breakfast all become easier as you adjust.

You can find recipes for many of these options online. In addition, *Paleo Cookbook For Dummies* by Kellyann Petrucci (Wiley) has a range of recipes for all your Paleo munching needs.

Milk Chocolate for Dark Chocolate

Cacao beans are basically nature's magic bullets. They're massively high in antioxidants — so high, in fact, that the top three sources of antioxidants in nature are from the cacao plant! But the more processed chocolate is, the fewer of these antioxidants you get. Milk chocolate is high in sugar and most often contains milk solids and soy. Dark chocolate with a minimum of 70 percent cacao solids is a much better option and a rich treat for anyone thriving on a Paleo lifestyle. In fact, the darker the chocolate the better!

High-cacao dark chocolate gets its characteristic rich, bitter, delicious flavor from all the minerals, powerful antioxidants, and healthy fats that give it true superfood status. After you've gotten used to switching out milk chocolate for dark chocolate, you'll discover a whole host of flavors hidden beneath those top notes and find out why chocolate truly is a sensual experience as you savor the silky texture. So next time you go shopping, grab a bar of high-cacao dark chocolate and enjoy the delicious taste of good health!

Add raw cacao powder to smoothies and coffee. Sprinkle cookies, muffins, and other desserts with raw cacao nibs for added antioxidants.

Peanut Butter for Seed, Nut, or Coconut Butters

Peanut butter is certainly delicious, but peanuts are technically a legume and therefore aren't particularly Paleo-friendly. To satisfy your peanut butter cravings, eat almond, cashew, or hazelnut butter instead. In fact, you can turn any of your favorite nuts into to smooth, creamy butters and enjoy them as spreads or by the spoonful. Simply add the nuts to your food processor or high speed blender and process until you achieve the right consistency. You can also buy an array of premade nut butters in grocery stores.

Sunflower seed butter tastes almost identical to natural peanut butter. In fact, when you use sunflower seed butter in baked goods in place of peanut butter, your product will taste just like it would if you had used peanut butter. Sunflower seed butter is readily available in most health food stores, or you can grind up your own in a food processor.

For a nut-free and seed-free alternative to peanut butter, use coconut butter. Coconut butter tastes different from nut and seed butters, but it has that same delicious creaminess and it's incredibly good for you!

Water for Bone Broth

Bone broth is one of the most nutritious and healing Paleo foods that should be part of any healthy diet. Swapping water for bone broth when making soups, sauces, or cooking vegetables is a great and inexpensive way to enhance the taste of food while boosting your intake of essential minerals such as calcium, magnesium, and phosphorus, which help to improve bone and tooth health. Bone broth also strengthens the immune system and aids in digestion. Because it's made from bones, it's high in collagen and supports healthy joints, hair, skin, and nails. The collagen comes from the joints and skin as opposed to the bone marrow, and it's so powerful that when you consume it, it strengthens your own connective tissue, smoothing your skin and even helping eliminate cellulite from the body.

You can make homemade bone broth from the bones of beef, bison, lamb, poultry, or fish. Whenever possible, ensure you're using high quality bones from pasture-raised animals or wild-caught fish. Simply cover the bones with water, add a small amount of vinegar or lemon juice, and allow it to cook at low heat for several hours. Cooking time varies. Beef bones can be cooked for over 24 hours; chicken bones take less time, about 10 to 15 hours.

Using a slow cooker to make bone broth is a great idea because you can turn the machine to low, set the desired time, and let it cook while you're away.

Pasta for Zucchini or Squash Noodles

For a healthier meal choice, enjoy zucchini or squash noodles as a delicious substitute for pasta. Using affordable vegetable peelers such as a spiral slicer or julienne peeler, you can transform these delicious vegetables into fettuccini, spaghetti, or even lasagna noodles.

Zucchini and squash noodles have a fantastic noodle-like texture and a mild flavor. Coupled with your favorite Paleo-friendly pasta sauce, they taste amazing and add to the nutritional content of your meals. Cooking the veggie noodles is as simple as steaming, roasting, microwaving, or sautéing them with your favorite spices.

Soy Sauce for Coconut Aminos

The perfect Paleo alternative to soy sauce is coconut aminos. *Coconut aminos* are a naturally aged blend of sea salt and the sap extracted from the coconut tree; they taste very similar to soy sauce, and you can use them in Asian-inspired meals, as a dipping sauce, or for salad dressings and marinades. Coconut aminos contain 17 essential amino acids, are rich in minerals, and are *low-glycemic* (meaning they have a slower, more desirable impact on your blood sugar). You can find them at health food stores. My brand of choice is Coconut Secret.

Rice for Cauliflower Rice

It may sound strange, but the best Paleo substitute for rice is cauliflower. Supplementing your meals with *riced* (finely grated) cauliflower is a simple way to give your body a boost of nutrients.

You can use your food processor (my preferred method) or cheese grater to grate the cauliflower head into small grains. The smaller the grains, the better the texture and the more quickly it cooks, so make sure to use the small teeth on your ricer of choice.

My favorite way to season my cauliflower rice is by adding a tablespoon of lime juice, ¼ cup of coconut milk, and fresh cilantro and salt to taste. Sauté the rice in coconut oil for about 20 minutes and serve. So easy and delicious!

Wheat-Based Pizza Crust for Paleo Pizza Crust

Did you know that you can still enjoy pizza on the Paleo diet? Making pizza crust with almond flour, cauliflower, or even broccoli gives you all of the pleasure of eating pizza without all the guilt.

Believe it or not, cauliflower makes for the most delicious and nutritious pizza crust. Making this crust does take some time, but it's worth the effort and is great to share with friends who don't believe eating Paleo can still be incredibly delicious. Using almond flour is a quicker way to make a Paleo pizza crust. Top your Paleo crust with your favorite pizza toppings, such as tomatoes, pepperoni, ham, pineapple, onions, olives, or raw cheese and enjoy one of the world's most savory foods without guilt.

Wheat and Corn Wraps for Paleo Wraps

Love burritos or sandwich wraps? So do most people around the world. Traditional wraps are typically wheat- or corn-based, but you can easily find alternatives that won't leave you feeling sluggish or bloated after you eat. Creating wholesome wraps with leafy greens is easy and delicious. Lettuce, cabbage, chard, collard greens, and kale make for great wraps that you can fill with your favorite foods.

Another option is homemade Paleo tortillas. These wraps are usually made with coconut flour; eggs, butter, or coconut oil; and sometimes a starch such as tapioca flour. Some recipes also use flaxseed meal to make the wrap taste more like the original wheat-based tortilla. Paleo tortillas are perfect for making breakfast burritos and sandwich wraps. You can also use them as crêpes filled with savory sweets such as fruits, whipped cream, and chocolate.

Traditional Breakfast Foods (Or No Breakfast) for Whole Foods

Breakfast is the most important meal of the day. It sets the tone for whether you'll be productive and energized or hungry, sluggish, and mentally out of sorts. Many people are used to starting their mornings with grains, pastries, a cup of sweetened coffee, or no food at all, but these foods cause blood sugar spikes that trigger food cravings and eventually weight gain and various health conditions. (And don't even get me started on the perils of skipping breakfast altogether. Even those who aren't hungry in the morning can benefit from the stable energy levels a Paleo breakfast provides.)

Transitioning to eating *whole foods* (unprocessed foods with no additives or artificial substances) for breakfast can be very difficult. You may even be asking "If I can't have cereal/donuts/pancakes, what's left?" Answer: Eggs, bacon, sausage, avocado, non-starchy veggies, coconut milk, berries, and even leftover steak or salmon make great, healthy breakfast options. The key is that you eat a nutrient-dense breakfast high in healthy fats and protein and low in sugars. (*Nutrient density* refers to how many nutrients a food contains relative to how many calories it contains.) Of course, you can also have Paleo toast, bagels, burritos, muffins, pancakes, and waffles on special occasions.

Cook your eggs in bacon fat, lard, coconut oil, or pastured butter to increase the nutrient and fat content of your meal. If smoothies are your breakfast of choice, add coconut milk, coconut oil, chia seeds, and leafy green vegetables for a Paleo powerhouse.

Energy and Sports Drinks for Coconut Water

Whether you're a serious Paleo athlete performing at a top level or just take long walks on the beach, your body needs some replenishment after physical activity. Rehydrate yourself naturally by drinking coconut water in place of energy drinks and sports drinks. Coconut water is a superfood that's not only rich in vitamins and minerals but also contains electrolytes that rehydrate you and give you a boost of energy. It increases your metabolism, keeps your heart in healthy shape, and keeps your skin looking young and vibrant. Sports drinks, on the other hand, are chemically engineered concoctions that contain sugars, sodium, toxic artificial dyes, and mysterious "natural flavors."

Coconut water is sold in most grocery stores in cans or bottles. Look for brands that have coconut water as the only ingredient. A better option is to drink the water directly from the nut, so check your local store to see if they carry real coconuts.

In addition to coconut water, try other natural sports drinks such as Kefir and Kombucha, or mix Vitamin C powder with water and your favorite fruit juice.

Index

• C •

• N •

Notes

Notes

Notes

Notes

Notes

Notes

About the Author

Adriana Harlan has literally transformed desserts into delicious, healthy, and nourishing treats. Along the way she's become one of the top healthy-dessert chefs in the world. She's the author of the award-winning blog *Living Healthy with Chocolate* (www.livinghealthywithchocolate.com), where she shares new recipes and wellness tips weekly. Her recipes have been featured in a number of Paleo and gluten-free magazines and blogs around the globe.

For most of her life, Adriana struggled with sugar cravings that were impossible to control. In her late 20s, she began suffering from debilitating stomach cramps and crippling joint pain that threatened to derail her athletic career and even rob her of her mobility. Several visits to various doctors brought no answers or relief. She was desperate to find a solution, but was confused about what exactly *healthy foods* were, and ultimately which foods would best nurture and heal her body. Having a degree in Biology, she used her scientific background to dig deep into numerous scientific studies and books in search of a solution. Adriana began to understand what was causing the inflammation in her body and has followed a strict Paleo diet since early 2010. Not long after, she felt better and was able to regain her health. But there was one thing she really missed — desserts. One day, she decided, "There must be dessert, too!" She discovered a whole new world of nutritious ingredients in nuts, seeds, cacao, coconut, and natural sweeteners like raw honey, and she began developing recipes.

Today with the knowledge Adriana has, she is inspired to guide you to improve your lives and achieve your health goals. Through her dessert recipes Adriana expresses her love for real whole foods and teaches you step by step how simple, wholesome, nutrient-rich ingredients can be combined to create delicious, healthy treats.

You can follow Adriana on her blog at www.livinghealthywith chocolate.com, and get new recipes and wellness tips to begin creating the healthy body and life you love.

Dedication

I want to dedicate this book to my husband and best friend Chuck. Without your patience and extensive support for the last 15 years I would not be where I am today. And to my mom Elizabeth and brother Alexandre who are constantly helping me grow and succeed at everything I do. I love each of you with all my heart.

Acknowledgements

First, I want to give a special thanks to all the readers on my blog at Living Healthy With Chocolate. Your comments, feedback, and support brought me to where I am today, put me on the path to writing this book, and I am extremely grateful to all of you. Your feedback on my recipes has been inspiring and humbling, and has changed my life!

A heartfelt thanks goes to my neighbors Scott and Susan Valle, and to all my friends who are my weekly taste testers. Your feedback on my recipes has been invaluable!

Thank you Chris Martino for gifting me with *Deep Nutrition* by Dr. Cate Shanaham, one of the greatest health books I have read. Reading this book changed the course of my life forever.

I want to thank the Paleo community of bloggers, researchers, functional medicine doctors, and the media for helping to change the lives of people through nutrition. You all have played a role in changing my life and health, and I'm forever grateful. It's because of your passion and hard work that the health of so many thousands of people has improved.

Finally, I want to thank my editors Tracy Boggier and Susan Hobbs for believing in me and helping me make writing a cookbook a dream come true. To arts and permission researcher Alicia South at John Wiley & Sons, thank you for allowing me to photograph the recipes in this cookbook.

Publisher's Acknowledgments

Acquisitions Editor: Tracy Boggier

Project Editor: Susan Hobbs

Copy Editor: Megan Knoll

Technical Editors: Katie Haldeman

Art Coordinator: Alicia B. South

Production Editor: Vinitha Vikraman

Project Manager: Jennifer Ehrlich

Cover Image: ©Adriana Harlan

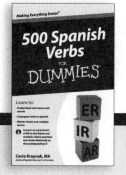
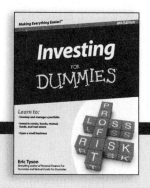 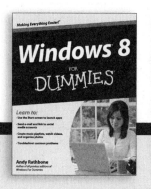 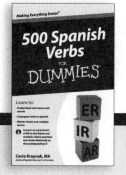 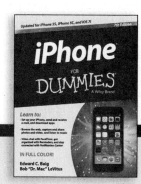

Math & Science

Algebra I For Dummies,
2nd Edition
978-0-470-55964-2

Anatomy and Physiology
For Dummies, 2nd Edition
978-0-470-92326-9

Astronomy For Dummies,
3rd Edition
978-1-118-37697-3

Biology For Dummies,
2nd Edition
978-0-470-59875-7

Chemistry For Dummies,
2nd Edition
978-1-118-00730-3

1001 Algebra II Practice
Problems For Dummies
978-1-118-44662-1

Microsoft Office

Excel 2013 For Dummies
978-1-118-51012-4

Office 2013 All-in-One
For Dummies
978-1-118-51636-2

PowerPoint 2013
For Dummies
978-1-118-50253-2

Word 2013 For Dummies
978-1-118-49123-2

Music

Blues Harmonica
For Dummies
978-1-118-25269-7

Guitar For Dummies,
3rd Edition
978-1-118-11554-1

iPod & iTunes
For Dummies, 10th Edition
978-1-118-50864-0

Programming

Beginning Programming
with C For Dummies
978-1-118-73763-7

Excel VBA Programming
For Dummies, 3rd Edition
978-1-118-49037-2

Java For Dummies,
6th Edition
978-1-118-40780-6

Religion & Inspiration

The Bible For Dummies
978-0-7645-5296-0

Buddhism For Dummies,
2nd Edition
978-1-118-02379-2

Catholicism For Dummies,
2nd Edition
978-1-118-07778-8

Self-Help & Relationships

Beating Sugar Addiction
For Dummies
978-1-118-54645-1

Meditation For Dummies,
3rd Edition
978-1-118-29144-3

Seniors

Laptops For Seniors
For Dummies, 3rd Edition
978-1-118-71105-7

Computers For Seniors
For Dummies, 3rd Edition
978-1-118-11553-4

iPad For Seniors
For Dummies, 6th Edition
978-1-118-72826-0

Social Security
For Dummies
978-1-118-20573-0

Smartphones & Tablets

Android Phones
For Dummies, 2nd Edition
978-1-118-72030-1

Nexus Tablets
For Dummies
978-1-118-77243-0

Samsung Galaxy S 4
For Dummies
978-1-118-64222-1

Samsung Galaxy Tabs
For Dummies
978-1-118-77294-2

Test Prep

ACT For Dummies,
5th Edition
978-1-118-01259-8

ASVAB For Dummies,
3rd Edition
978-0-470-63760-9

GRE For Dummies,
7th Edition
978-0-470-88921-3

Officer Candidate Tests
For Dummies
978-0-470-59876-4

Physician's Assistant Exam
For Dummies
978-1-118-11556-5

Series 7 Exam For Dummies
978-0-470-09932-2

Windows 8

Windows 8.1 All-in-One
For Dummies
978-1-118-82087-2

Windows 8.1 For Dummies
978-1-118-82121-3

Windows 8.1 For Dummies,
Book + DVD Bundle
978-1-118-82107-7

Available in print and e-book formats.

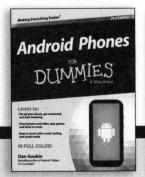
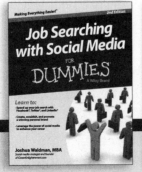
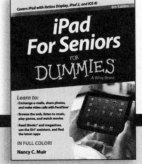
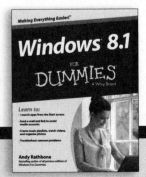

Available wherever books are sold. **For more information or to order direct visit www.dummies.com**

Take Dummies with you everywhere you go!

Whether you are excited about e-books, want more from the web, must have your mobile apps, or are swept up in social media, Dummies makes everything easier.

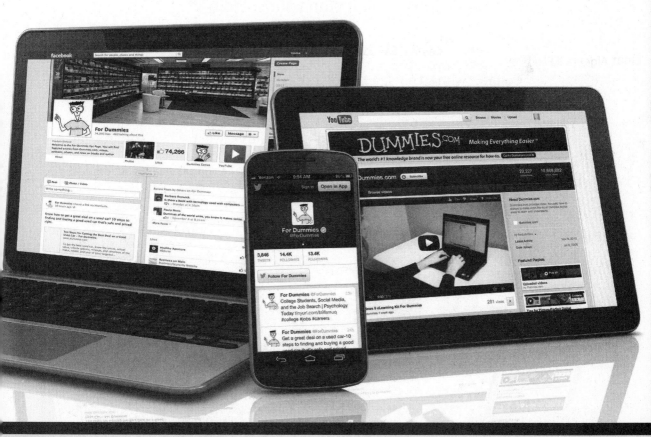

For Dummies is the global leader in the reference category and one of the most trusted and highly regarded brands in the world. No longer just focused on books, customers now have access to the For Dummies content they need in the format they want. Let us help you develop a solution that will fit your brand and help you connect with your customers.

Advertising & Sponsorships

Connect with an engaged audience on a powerful multimedia site, and position your message alongside expert how-to content.

Targeted ads • Video • Email marketing • Microsites • Sweepstakes sponsorship

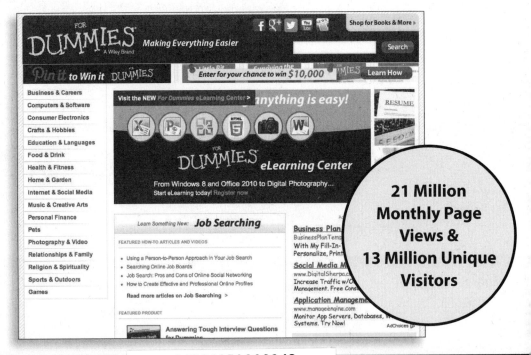

31901056260948

Custom Publishing

Reach a global audience in any language by creating a solution that will differentiate you from competitors, amplify your message, and encourage customers to make a buying decision.

Apps • Books • eBooks • Video • Audio • Webinars

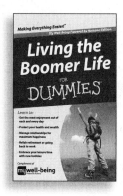
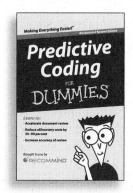
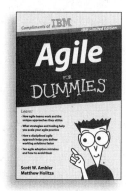
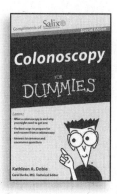

Brand Licensing & Content

Leverage the strength of the world's most popular reference brand to reach new audiences and channels of distribution.

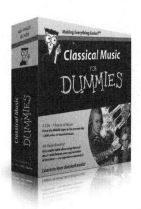
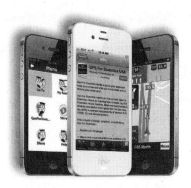
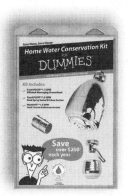
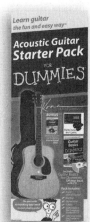

For more information, visit www.Dummies.com/biz

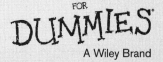

Dummies products make life easier!

- DIY
- Consumer Electronics
- Crafts

- Software
- Cookware
- Hobbies

- Videos
- Music
- Games
- and More!

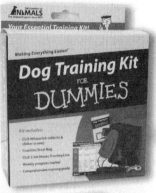

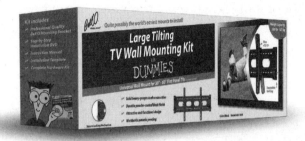

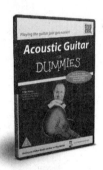

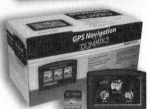

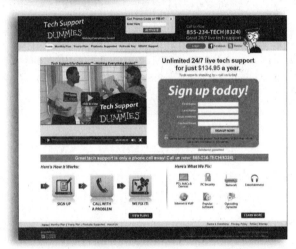

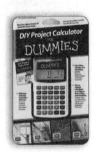

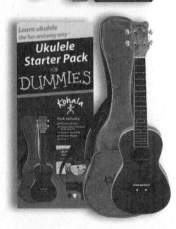

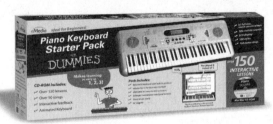

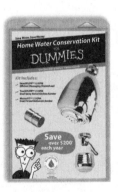

For more information, go to **Dummies.com** and search the store by category.

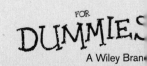